Multiple-choice Questions in Clinical Gastroenterology

Cardiac Intensive Care.
Morriston

Other Examination Preparation Books Published by Petroc Press:

Multiple-choice Questions in Clinical Gastroenterology

Malcolm C. Bateson (Editor)

Consultant Physician and Gastroenterologist
General Hospital, Bishop Auckland, County Durham, UK

and

Twenty-three Teachers

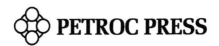 PETROC PRESS

Petroc Press, an imprint of Librapharm Limited

Distributors

Plymbridge Distributors Limited, Plymbridge House, Estover Road, Plymouth PL6 7PZ, UK

Published in the United Kingdom by LibraPharm Limited, 3 Thames Court, High Street, Goring-on-Thames, Reading, Berkshire RG8 9AR, UK

A catalogue record for this book is available from the British Library

ISBN 1 900603 51 9

Typeset by
Richard Powell Editorial and Production Services, Basingstoke, Hampshire
Printed and bound in the United Kingdom by
BPC Wheatons, Hennock Road, Marsh Barton, Exeter, Devon, EX2 8RP

Contents

Preface

In the middle of the twelfth century the Scottish Sovereign's rule extended into England north of the River Tees. The territory of this ancient kingdom of Caledonia is today an area where the National Health Service functions best and academic medicine flourishes. Gastroenterology is particularly strong and so it is especially appropriate that colleagues from north Britain contribute to this collection of multiple-choice questions (MCQs).

These MCQs focus on common clinical problems approached in different ways and on recent advances. Many are based on real patients under the clinical care of the authors. Often detailed explanations of the answers are provided.

The questions are of varying levels of difficulty so as to be suitable for all levels of medical postgraduates.

MCQs should only be attempted if the correct answer is definitely known or almost certain. Not only do wrong answers lose marks, but also they may be falsely remembered as 'facts'.

The strength of this book lies in the experience and merits of the authors. The editor accepts all blame for any problems!

Authors

M. C. Bateson (*Editor*)	Bishop Auckland General Hospital
R. G. Barton	North Tyneside General Hospital
D. Burke	Cumberland Infirmary, Carlisle
P. Cann	South Cleveland Hospital, Middlesborough
J. Cox	Wansbeck Hospital, Northumberland
G. Curry	Gartnavel General Hospital, Glasgow
S. Ghosh	Western General Hospital, Edinburgh
W. S. Hislop	Royal Alexandra Hospital, Paisley
D. Hopwood	Ninewells Hospital, Dundee
D. Johnston	Ninewells Hospital, Dundee
Alison L. Jones	Edinburgh Royal Infirmary
Sarah L. Jowett	Royal Sunderland Hospital
A. F. Macklon	North Durham Hospitals
K. Matthewson	Hexham General Hospital
J. O'Donohue	Gartnavel General Hospital, Glasgow
K. R. Palmer	Western General Hospital, Edinburgh
T. Reilly	Victoria Infirmary, Glasgow
J. D. R. Rose	Ayr Hospital
N. Sivaramakrishnan	Sunderland Royal Hospital
Heather Smith	Bishop Auckland General Hospital
J. G. Stephen	Bishop Auckland General Hospital
P. N. Trewby	Darlington Memorial Hospital
J. Wilson	Victoria Hospital, Kirkcaldy
R. A. B. Wood	Ninewells Hospital, Dundee

1. Nutrition, Mouth, Pharynx and Oesophagus

Q1.1 **Drugs which are effective in gastro-oesophageal reflux disease are:**

A. Astemizole
B. Lansoprazole
C. Mebendazole
D. Omeprazole
E. Pantoprazole

Q1.2 **A 62-year-old man with a past right hemiplegia complains of increasing dysphagia for solids over a period of three months. His weight is steady.**

A. This will be explained by cerebrovascular disease and no investigations are necessary
B. Gastroscopy is the logical test
C. Barium swallow may show aspiration of contrast
D. If there is a stricture endoscopic dilatation will help the problem
E. Percutaneous endoscopic gastrostomy is needed

Q1.3 **Vitamin B12 in diet:**

A. Binds to intrinsic factor in the stomach
B. May be inadequate in vegetarians
C. Requires adequate pancreatic function for absorption
D. Is transported into portal circulation bound to R protein
E. Is poorly absorbed during pregnancy

Q1.4 **Obese individuals (compared with lean subjects):**

A. Absorb more calories from their food
B. Have a greater energy expenditure
C. Have a higher incidence of hypertension
D. Carry excess body tissue which consists of 50% fat and 50% non-fat tissue
E. With excess abdominal fat (android obesity) are at greater risk of diabetes and atheroma than those with peripheral (gynaecoid) obesity

Q1.5   Oesophageal carcinoma is very common in:

A. Iran
B. Romania
C. China
D. Northern Ireland
E. Tasmania

Q1.6   In achalasia of the cardia:

A. The diagnosis may be suggested by the chest x-ray
B. Peristalsis is normal in the dilated oesophagus above the narrowed lower end
C. Odynophagia (painful swallowing) may be a symptom
D. Recurrent respiratory infections may be the presenting feature
E. Muscle relaxants are the treatment of choice

Q1.7   A 70-year-old cigarette smoking man presents with dysphagia for solids. At endoscopy a stricture is apparent in the distal oesophagus. Cytology shows squamous atypical cells:

A. Benign reflux stricture is almost certainly the cause
B. Adenocarcinoma of Barrett's oesophagus is much more likely than squamous carcinoma
C. CT scanning is better than endosonography in staging tumour
D. Laser therapy and radiotherapy have important roles in treatment
E. Total parenteral nutrition is commonly used

Q1.8   Combination chemoradiotherapy for oesophageal carcinoma:

A. Should be considered for most patients
B. Is particularly useful in unresectable squamous carcinoma
C. Consists of x-ray treatment plus drugs such as cisplatin and fluorouracil
D. Improves 5-year survival over radiotherapy alone
E. Is too expensive for wide use

Q1.9   Raised serum folate levels are seen in:

A. Coeliac disease
B. Epilepsy
C. Spina bifida
D. Bacterial overgrowth of the small bowel
E. Alcoholism

Q1.10 Achalasia of the oesophagus:

A. Is thought to have a strong genetic basis
B. Can be reliably discriminated from pseudo-achalasia due to malignant tumours by oesophageal manometric features
C. Is characterised by dysphagia to liquids rather than solids
D. Is associated with degenerative changes in the vagal dorsal motor nucleus
E. Most commonly presents in children

Q1.11 Raised serum ferritin levels are seen in:

A. Pernicious anaemia
B. Malignant disease
C. Acute illness
D. Iron deficiency anaemia
E. Haemochromatosis

Q1.12 Symptoms of gastro-oesophageal reflux include:

A. Chest pain
B. Breathlessness
C. Waterbrash
D. Hiccoughs
E. Chronic cough

Q1.13 B12 deficiency anaemia may indicate:

A. Dietary inadequacy
B. Auto-immune gastritis
C. Pancreatic insufficiency
D. Small bowel resection
E. Pernicious anaemia

Q1.14 Oral recurrent aphthous ulceration (RAU) is associated with:

A. Coeliac disease
B. Pancreatic disease
C. Diverticular disease
D. Crohn's disease
E. Iron deficiency

Q1.15 Barrett's oesophagus:

A. This condition indicates the presence of abnormal squamous epithelium in the distal oesophagus
B. If left untreated will cause carcinoma in around 50% of cases
C. If marked dysplasia is present then surgery is the only possible treatment
D. In order to detect a single asymptomatic cancer one will have to screen about 30 patients
E. Proton pump inhibitors (PPIs) will reliably cause distal migration of the squamocolumnar junction

Q1.16 In patients with oesophageal dysmotility due to achalasia:

A. Mortality is usually due to respiratory complications
B. Balloon dilatation is the recommended therapy
C. Botulinum toxin is effective as treatment
D. Medical treatments provide effective symptom relief in most patients
E. Surgical treatment of the achalasia usually requires anti-reflux procedures

Q1.17 In diffuse oesophageal spasm:

A. Intermittent, simultaneous oesophageal contractions are interspersed with normal swallow-induced peristalsis
B. Relaxation of the lower oesophageal sphincter is normal
C. The diagnosis may be made by observation of tertiary contractions on barium swallow
D. Nitrates may reduce the symptoms
E. Cardiomyotomy (Heller's myotomy) is recommended

Q1.18 A 50-year-old man presents complaining of heartburn but no dysphagia. His endoscopy shows mild (Savary-Miller Grade 1) oesophagitis. You explain your findings and discuss therapeutic options with him:

A. Antral gastritis has no relevance to the occurrence of his gastro-oesophageal reflux
B. *Helicobacter* eradication will increase the likelihood that long-term medication for gastro-oesophageal reflux will not be necessary
C. *Helicobacter* eradication increases the likelihood that acid suppression therapy will be successful in controlling his symptoms
D. Therapy which successfully resolves his symptoms will reliably heal his oesophagus also
E. Anti-reflux surgery has a mortality of 0.5%

Q1.19 Which of the following occur with achalasia of the cardia?

A. Initial difficulty in swallowing solids but not liquids
B. Severe spontaneous retrosternal pain relieved by drinking cold water
C. Initial rapid and severe weight loss
D. Retrosternal impact pain within 10 seconds of the swallowing
E. Increased incidence of squamous carcinoma of the oesophagus

Q1.20 Oesophageal carcinoma:

A. Responds best to chemoradiation followed by radical surgery
B. Causes dermatomyositis
C. May follow oesophageal damage from corrosive ingestion
D. Complicates chronic gastro-oesophageal acid reflux
E. Is becoming less common in Western populations

Q1.21 Hypertensive oesophageal peristalsis (the 'nutcracker oesophagus'):

A. Is defined by oesophageal-body primary peristaltic waves with amplitude peaks of > 250 mmHg
B. The normal pattern of aboral progression of the oesophageal-body contraction is preserved
C. Often presents clinically as the globus sensation
D. May produce dysphagia
E. Responds to treatment with beta-adrenergic antagonists

Q1.22 A 14-year-old boy ingested 500 ml of bleach as a dare. You see evidence of oropharyngeal ulceration on examination and he has a hoarse voice:

A. His severity of injury can be predicted from knowledge of the volume and concentration of bleach ingested
B. His oropharyngeal and laryngeal injury predict the existence of oesophageal injury
C. Prompt endoscopy is required
D. Grey or brown/black ulceration at endoscopy suggest transmural injury
E. Oesophageal stricture is prevented by routine dilatation in the first two weeks after injury

Q1.23 Treatment of the following causes of infective oesophagitis is appropriate with the following agents:

A. Varicella zoster in an immunocompetent patient with acyclovir
B. Cytomegalovirus (CMV) in an immunocompromised patient with foscarnet
C. Tuberculosis (TB) with erythromycin
D. Candida in an immunocompromised patient with nystatin
E. Herpes simplex in an immunocompromised patient with foscarnet

Q1.24 Barrett's oesophagus:

A. Is a dysplastic change of the oesophageal squamous epithelium
B. Progressively extends up the oesophagus if untreated
C. Is associated with reflux oesophagitis
D. Occurs more often in men than women
E. In otherwise fit patients, should be treated by oesophagectomy

Q1.25 Achalasia:

A. Is due to impaired inhibitory innervation of the oesophagus
B. Characteristically shows preservation of normal oesophageal body peristalsis
C. Has a peak incidence in patients aged 30–40 years
D. May occur as a paraneoplastic neural dysfunction
E. May be treated by injection of botulinum toxin

Q1.26 A 70-year-old man complains that he regurgitates food eaten some hours previously unaltered. He has no dysphagia. The likely diagnosis is:

A. Achalasia of the cardia
B. Cricopharyngeal achalasia
C. Zenker's diverticulum
D. Carcinoma of the mid-thoracic oesophagus
E. Rolling hiatus hernia

Q1.27 A man 26-year-old with no previous gastrointestinal symptoms and who is known to abuse alcohol was admitted with a haematemesis after an alcoholic binge. Gastroscopy shows oesophagitis and two clean Mallory–Weiss tears. The haemoglobin level is 135 g/l. Appropriate management might include:

A. Same day discharge
B. Treatment with H2 blockade
C. Treatment with proton pump inhibitor
D. Observation overnight and discharge the following day
E. Adrenaline injection to reduce the incidence of rebleeding

Q1.28 A heterosexual 19-year-old man is admitted following a haematemesis. Gastroscopy reveals oesophageal varices. He drinks regularly but not to excess. His past medical history includes an interval appendicectomy. His prothrombin time and liver biopsy are normal. Which of the following investigations are most likely to be helpful in making a diagnosis:

A. Liver biopsy
B. Hepatitis B serology
C. Ferritin level
D. Colour Doppler ultrasound
E. Portography

Q1.29 In gastro-oesophageal reflux disease:

A. The diagnosis is reliably excluded by a normal endoscopy
B. Symptoms correlate well with the severity of the endoscopic findings
C. Proton pump inhibitors control the symptoms well but are ineffective at healing oesophagitis
D. After completion of a satisfactory course of proton pump inhibitors symptomatic relapse is uncommon
E. Long-term proton pump inhibitor treatment reduces the likelihood of stricture recurrence after successful dilatation

Q1.30 A 60-year-old man has an oesophagectomy for Barrett's oesophagus complicated by adenocarcinoma of the oesophagus of the distal third at another hospital. He is admitted with repeated vomiting since the operation associated with a two stone weight loss. Gastroscopy shows no mucosal abnormality. What treatment would be most likely to improve him:

A. Proton pump inhibitors
B. Proton pump inhibitors and cisapride
C. Psychotherapy and cancer counselling
D. CT scan of head for a posterior fossa secondary
E. Pyloroplasty and drainage procedure

Q1.31 A 50-year-old man goes on an alcoholic binge and has an episode of severe vomiting at home. He later presents to Casualty with severe epigastric pain radiating to the back. He is found to be very ill. His amylase and ECG are normal, and a chest x-ray shows a pleural effusion. What diagnosis would be most likely:

A. Acute pancreatitis
B. Perforated duodenal ulcer
C. Mallory–Weiss tear
D. Boerhaave's syndrome
E. Gastric volvulus

Q1.32 In Barrett's oesophagus:

A. The risk of developing oesophageal cancer is approximately four times that of the normal population
B. The risk of developing oesophageal cancer is related to the presence of intestinal as opposed to gastric metaplasia
C. Endoscopic screening programmes have been shown to improve the mortality from oesophageal cancer
D. Long-term treatment with proton pump inhibitors allows complete resolution of the columnar metaplasia
E. Early oesophageal cancer can be reliably excluded by careful endoscopic inspection of the mucosa

Q1.33 Oesophageal varices:

A. Variceal bleeding, if not treated prophylactically, is an inevitable outcome in cirrhosis of the liver
B. Oesophageal varices should routinely be treated prophylactically with injection sclerotherapy
C. Beta-blockade is shown to reduce the risk of a first bleeding episode from oesophageal varices
D. Endoscopic band ligation of varices is as at least as effective as sclerotherapy in preventing rebleeding
E. Overall 2-year mortality in cirrhotic patients with varices is not affected by any variceal treatment modality.

Q1.34 A 72-year-old man with a metastatic adenocarcinoma of the lower oesophagus has a stent placed in March of this year. He returns, however, in August with painless dysphagia:

A. The likeliest cause is food bolus obstruction
B. Barium swallow should be done as a first investigation
C. A second stent may be required
D. This carcinoma is not suitable for radiotherapy management
E. He will require referral to a unit with fulguration or laser facilities

Q1.35 In a patient with an Hb of 7.0 g/dl, MCHC 23%, MCV 69 fl and MCH 26 pg:

A. The anaemia is unlikely to be caused by menstrual loss in females under age 45
B. The patient may have blue sclerae
C. Such a blood picture may be associated with pica
D. The patient should normally receive a blood transfusion
E. Beta-thalassaemia needs to be considered

Q1.36 Malabsorption of vitamin B12 may occur under the following conditions:

A. Treatment with acid secretory inhibitors
B. Treatment with beta-blockers
C. Vegetarianism
D. Imerslund-Grasbeck syndrome
E. Chronic pancreatitis

Q1.37 In a patient presenting with weight loss:

A. $\dfrac{\text{Weight (kg)}}{\text{Height (m)}}$ is a useful index
B. Parenteral nutrition is the most appropriate intervention to reverse weight loss
C. Petechiae may be a sign of vitamin C deficiency
D. Modified enteral nutrition may be effective as a primary therapy in small bowel Crohn's disease
E. An accurate dietary history is essential

Q1.38 In a 36-year-old male presenting with a symptom of heartburn:

A. Endoscopy is essential
B. Lifestyle changes may significantly improve symptoms
C. *H. pylori* (Hp) eradication is likely to improve symptoms
D. Proton pump inhibitors should be prescribed as a first line therapy
E. Endoscopic features of oesophageal reflux are invariably present

Q1.39 In morbid obesity:

A. Longevity is not diminished
B. BMI is greater than 40
C. Reducing diets are futile
D. Serum leptin concentration is decreased
E. There is increased incidence of pulmonary embolism

Q1.40 A 54-year-old man gives a year history of gradually worsening painless dysphagia and weight loss of 2 stones. He has been waking at night with a cough for 6 months. He is a smoker:

A. Bronchial carcinoma, invading the oesophagus, is the most likely diagnosis
B. Peptic oesophageal stricturing is not unusual in the absence of a story of pain or heartburn
C. Achalasia is characterised by powerful oesophageal peristalsis with failure of the lower oesophageal sphincter to relax
D. Adenocarcinoma of the oesophagus has a better prognosis for survival than squamous carcinoma of the oesophagus
E. A diagnosis of achalasia is compatible with entirely normal appearance at endoscopy

1. Answers

A1.1
A. False
B. True
C. False
D. True
E. True
Lansoprazole, omeprazole and pantoprazole are proton pump inhibitor (PPI) gastric acid anti-secretory drugs of equal efficacy. Astemizole is a non-sedating anti-histamine and mebendazole is an anti-helminth agent.

A1.2
A. False
B. True
C. True
D. True
E. False
Although cerebrovascular disease can cause dysphagia other diagnoses need to be considered. There could be either a benign or malignant oesophageal stricture. Gastroscopy will permit macroscopic diagnosis, cytology and histology, and it also offers the possibility of therapeutic dilation. Aspiration of x-ray contrast is a risk in pharyngeal inco-ordination, but many radiologists prefer to use dilute barium rather than water-soluble iodine contrast because of superior images.

A1.3
A. False
B. True
C. True
D. False
E. False
Dietary vitamin B12 is mainly derived from animal sources and most vegetables are poor in vitamin B12 content. Vitamin B12 is released from dietary proteins by gastric acid and binds to R protein secreted in saliva. Intrinsic factor secreted in the stomach has a much lower affinity for vitamin B12 than R protein and can only bind to the vitamin in the duodenum after the R protein is hydrolysed by pancreatic trypsin. The intrinsic factor–vitamin B12 complex resists proteolysis and reaches the terminal ileum to bind to specific receptors on the ileal enterocytes.

Vitamin B12 absorption doubles during pregnancy as the number of receptors increases. The intrinsic factor–vitamin B12 complex enters the cell by translocation, is split up within the enterocytes and free vitamin B12 (cobalamin) leaves the cell bound to ileal transcobalamin II which transports it into the portal circulation.

A1.4
A. False
B. True
C. True
D. False
E. True

Many studies have shown that both lean and obese people absorb approximately 95% of the energy which they ingest. The total energy loss in the faeces is about 5% of the intake. Experiments show that total energy expenditure is greater in obese than in lean subjects. The excess tissue response for increase in body weight over the ideal weight consists of roughly 75% fat and 25% fat-free tissue. The distribution of body fat appears to affect the morbidity associated with obesity. The waist/hip ratio has a greater predictive power for coronary heart disease than body mass index (BMI).

A1.5
A. True
B. False
C. True
D. False
E. False

There is a very high rate in the countries around the Caspian littoral (Iran and the southern republics of the former USSR) and also in Eastern China.

A1.6
A. True
B. False
C. True
D. True
E. False

A1.7
A. False
B. False
C. False
D. True
E. False

The evidence points to squamous carcinoma of the oesophagus. Biopsy histology should confirm this. Adenocarcinoma of the oesophagus is common but often reflects proximal growth of gastric carcinoma. Endosonography is better than magnetic resonance scanning, which is better than CT scanning in staging, but all of these may be proved wrong at thoracotomy. The object of treatment is to restore normal feeding as far as possible. Dilation and expanding metal stents placement also have useful roles.

A1.8
A. True
B. True
C. True
D. True
E. False

Where carcinoma is unsuitable for surgery, or even where adenocarcinoma can be operated upon, additional x-ray and drug treatment improves 5-year survival. Patients should be assessed for this treatment though it is not always appropriate.

A1.9
A. False
B. False
C. False
D. True
E. False

Small intestinal colonisation may be associated with bacterial folate synthesis (and vitamin B12 consumption). The other conditions have been linked with folate deficiency.

A1.10
A. False
B. False
C. False
D. True
E. False

Though the cause of achalasia is unknown, genetic influences are minimal. Onset of symptoms is generally in the third to fifth decades and less than 5% of patients have symptoms before adolescence. Loss of ganglion cells in the oesophageal wall and degenerative changes such as fragmentation and dissolution of the nuclear material in the dorsal motor nucleus of the vagus have been described. Dysphagia occurs with both liquids and solids. The differential diagnosis of most concern is a wide variety of malignant neoplasms presenting as pseudo-achalasia. CT scan and endoscopic ultrasound may distinguish the two conditions.

A1.11
A. False
B. True
C. True
D. False
E. True
Ferritin is both an acute phase protein and an indicator of body iron stores. It is low in iron deficiency anaemia. Elevated levels may be seen in malignant disease and any acute severe illness. Persistent markedly elevated levels suggest haemochromatosis which should be confirmed by liver biopsy.

A1.12
A. True
B. False
C. True
D. False
E. True
Reflux of acid into the oesophagus typically causes a burning chest pain with stimulation of salivary flow (waterbrash). Either reflexly or by direct irritation reflux can be a cause of cough. There is an association with asthma, but breathlessness should not be directly attributed to reflux.

A1.13
A. True
B. True
C. True
D. True
E. True

A1.14
A. True
B. False
C. False
D. True
E. True
RAU occurs predominantly as an isolated disorder but is increased in patients with a number of inflammatory gut diseases and also with deficiencies of iron, folic acid and vitamins.

A1.15
A. False
B. False
C. False
D. False
E. False

A1.16
A. True
B. True
C. True
D. False
E. True
Medical treatment for achalasia is only partially successful and is usually only a short-term measure. Balloon dilatation is effective in up to 75% of patients, and the recent use of botulinum toxin injected into the lower oesophageal sphincter has given similar results. After surgical myotomy the incidence of severe gastro-oesophageal reflux has led most surgeons to perform combined myotomy and anti-reflux surgery. Most deaths are due to aspiration.

A1.17
A. True
B. True
C. False
D. True
E. False
Occasional tertiary contractions may be seen on barium swallow in individuals without significant oesophageal disease and their presence does not establish a diagnosis of diffuse oesophageal spasm. The lower oesophageal sphincter functions normally in most patients and thus there is no indication for cardiomyotomy.

A1.18
A. True
B. False
C. False
D. False
E. True
Helicobacter eradication may increase intragastric acidity slightly and consequently may increase the requirement for anti-reflux medication. In symptomatic individuals, symptom resolution is a good predictor of oesophageal mucosal healing.

A1.19
A. False
B. True
C. False
D. True
E. False

A1.20
A. True
B. True
C. True
D. True
E. False

A1.21
A. True
B. True
C. False
D. False
E. False

The 'nutcracker oesophagus' may cause chest pain. It is characterised by high amplitude contractions with otherwise normal peristaltic progression. The contractions will be unaffected or may even be worsened by beta-adrenergic antagonists.

A1.22
A. False
B. False
C. True
D. True
E. False

Because of the relative lack of taste alkaline solutions are likely to be swallowed in larger amounts than acids. Alkaline injury is thus often very deep. The presence of oropharyngeal and laryngeal injury confirm that caustic ingestion has taken place but do not predict the existence or severity of oesophageal injury. Follow up for such patients should be by barium swallow at 2–3 weeks to screen for stricturing and then at three-monthly intervals for one year.

A1.23
A. True
B. True
C. False
D. False
E. True

Viral infection causing oesophagitis should be treated in either immuno-compromised or immunocompetent patients with antiviral agents. TB is not sensitive to erythromycin. Candida in an immunocompromised patient should be treated systemically with fluconazole rather than topically with nystatin.

A1.24
A. False
B. False
C. True
D. True
E. False

Barrett's oesophagus is a metaplastic change of the squamous epithelium in the oesophagus which is associated with reflux oesophagitis but shows little evidence of progressive extension. Oesophagectomy is only appropriate when the condition is complicated by high grade dysplasia or carcinoma.

A1.25
A. True
B. False
C. False
D. True
E. True

Achalasia may develop at any time in adult life and is associated with degeneration of the oesophageal myenteric plexus, particularly affecting the inhibitory innervation. Intra-sphincteric injection of botulinum toxin has recently been established as a safe treatment with moderate effectiveness.

A1.26
A. False
B. False
C. True
D. False
E. False

Zenker's diverticulum (a diverticulum arising from the posterior pharynx above the cricopharyngeus) causes such symptoms. Dysphagia is usually a late symptom indicating that the diverticulum has become large enough to swing distally and obstruct the upper oesophagus.

While patients with achalasia may regurgitate food, usually patients with achalasia complain of dysphagia. Cricopharyngeal achalasia may in a small percentage of patients relate to Zenker's diverticulum but does not cause regurgitation on its own.

A1.27
A. True
B. False
C. False
D. False
E. False

Oesophagitis with no symptoms should not lead to any treatment. Mallory–Weiss tears which are clean do not require any treatment and such patients are suitable for early discharge.

A1.28
A. False
B. False
C. False
D. True
E. True

This man presented late with an appendix mass and had an interval appendicectomy, at which time a portal vein thrombosis was found. He went on to develop portal hypertension. Colour Doppler ultrasound or portography would be the most helpful investigations. However, obtaining this man's lost hospital notes turned out to be the most useful 'procedure' here. After recurrent bleeds he had a very satisfactory shunt procedure.

A1.29
A. False
B. False
C. False
D. False
E. True

Only 70% of patients with symptomatic gastro-oesophageal reflux disease have oesophagitis visible at endoscopy and symptom severity correlates very poorly with the endoscopic findings. Proton pump inhibitors are effective controllers of symptoms and healers of oesophagitis, but symptoms usually relapse once they are discontinued.

A1.30
A. False
B. False
C. False
D. False
E. True
An oesophagectomy followed by persistent vomiting suggests that a drainage procedure has not been performed and such a patient will continue to vomit until he dies unless repeat surgery is performed. This patient did extremely well after his second surgical procedure.

A1.31
A. False
B. False
C. False
D. True
E. False
Boerhaave's syndrome is a rare condition but repeated vomiting followed by epigastric pain and the presence of a pleural effusion should suggest pressure rupture of the oesophagus (Boerhaave's syndrome). Pain on swallowing, breathlessness, occasionally hoarse voice and the findings of surgical emphysema of the neck, and the presence of a pleural effusion are all very suggestive.

A1.32
A. False
B. True
C. False
D. False
E. False
The risk of developing oesophageal cancer in Barrett's oesophagus patients is 40 times that of the normal population. Cardiac, gastric, intestinal and indeterminate types of metaplasia may develop with the increased risk of malignancy being within the latter two groups. There is no evidence that endoscopic screening reduces cancer mortality. Proton pump inhibition promotes the development of 'squamous islands' in the Barrett's oesophagus but not effective regression. The absence of any focal lesion on endoscopy does not exclude an early carcinoma.

A1.33
A. False
B. False
C. True
D. True
E. True

Only 33% of cirrhotic patients will bleed from oesophageal varices if left untreated. The Veterans' Administrations trial of sclerotherapy as primary prophylaxis reported in 1991 an increased mortality in the treatment arm. These two observations taken together mean that most clinicians would not offer primary sclerotherapy to unselected patients with oesophageal varices, although other trials have shown advantage in the treatment arm. Banding of varices has less potential to harm the oesophagus, is not contra-indicated when coagulopathy is present and has shown in several studies decreased rebleeding rates and morbidity, though not all-cause mortality, when compared with sclerotherapy. Its use as primary prophylaxis is currently under study. The routine use of beta-blockers where not contra-indicated is shown to prevent first bleeding.

A1.34
A. False
B. False
C. True
D. False
E. True

Adenocarcinoma of the oesophagus is more exophytic than squamous carcinoma of the oesophagus. Placement of stents will cause few problems with bolus obstruction. Tumour ingrowth in an uncovered stent or growth over either end of the stent, requires fulguration of the tumour and place-ment of a second stent partly inside the first stent. Radiotherapy can be used in adenocarcinoma and may delay further re-recurrence.

A1.35
A. False
B. True
C. True
D. False
E. True

Menstrual loss is by far the commonest cause of iron deficiency anaemia and can be presumed in the absence of any other symptoms. Iron deficiency anaemia can cause blue sclerae and pica and one would normally assess the response to iron before giving a blood transfusion. Beta-thalassaemia causes microcytic anaemia.

A1.36
A. True
B. False
C. False
D. True
E. True

There is evidence that H2 receptor antagonists and proton pump inhibitors decrease vitamin B12 absorption. Pancreatic exocrine insufficiency results in a lack of protease to release vitamin B12 from R protein, preventing absorption. Imerslund–Grasbeck syndrome is an autosomal recessive disorder of vitamin B12 malabsorption. Although vegetarian diets may be deficient in vitamin B12, any vitamin B12 present is absorbed normally.

A1.37
A. False
B. False
C. False
D. True
E. True

$$BMI\,(body\,mass\,index) = \frac{Weight\,(kg)}{Height^2\,(m)}$$

Parenteral nutrition should only be considered where there is a failure of gut function and not as a first line treatment for weight loss. Petechiae and ecchymoses are a sign of vitamin C deficiency. Enteral nutrition with elemental diet can be effective as a primary therapy of Crohn's disease. A dietary history is essential in cases of weight loss.

A1.38
A. False
B. True
C. False
D. False
E. False

Endoscopy would not be required unless the patient has worrying symptoms (i.e. weight loss, dysphagia, melaena, etc) and in many cases may be normal despite severe symptoms. Lifestyle changes (i.e. weight loss, stopping smoking, dietary modification, etc) plus antacids/alginates are often sufficient to improve symptoms, and potent anti-secretory drugs are best kept for patients not responding to such measures. There is no evidence that Hp eradication therapy improves reflux symptoms (and may indeed exacerbate them).

A1.39

A. False
B. True
C. True
D. False
E. True

Morbid obesity is a term which emphasises the morbidity associated with extreme obesity. Body mass index is a good measure of fatness. Most authorities define a morbidly obese individual as one with a BMI of more than 40. Whether or not obesity surgery is undertaken, life-long control of calorie intake is essential in a therapeutic strategy for morbid obesity. Extreme obesity impairs health and reduces longevity. The serum concentration of leptin (a protein produced by fat cells) is correlated with measures of obesity. A BMI of 29 and over is associated with a three-fold increase in the incidence of pulmonary embolism.

A1.40

A. False
B. True
C. False
D. False
E. True

Carcinoma is possible but unlikely with the long, gradually progressive history. There is a poor correlation between symptoms and endoscopic appearances of oesophagitis (including patients presenting with dysphagia). The pathognomonic feature of achalasia is the absence of oesophageal peristalsis, usually associated with poor sphincter relaxation. Endoscopy may be entirely normal in achalasia, although the retention of fluid or food within the oesophagus should alert the endoscopist.

2. Stomach, Duodenum, Gastrointestinal Bleeding and *Helicobacter pylori*

Q2.1 A fit 42-year-old man on no drugs is admitted with a bleeding duodenal ulcer. He gives a history of anti-*Helicobacter pylori* treatment in the past:

A. Re-investigation and re-treatment for *Helicobacter pylori* will be needed
B. The prior treatment for *Helicobacter pylori* is so effective it must have worked
C. Evaluation by IgG ELISA serology will indicate whether he carries *Helicobacter pylori*
D. Carbon-13 urea breath testing is likely to be positive
E. The disease may be fatal

Q2.2 Complications of peptic ulcer include:

A. Perforation
B. Haemorrhage
C. Gastric outflow obstruction
D. Pancreatitis
E. Jaundice

Q2.3 The use of non-steroidal anti-inflammatory drugs has led to an increase in:

A. Mouth ulcers
B. Oesophagitis
C. Gastric ulcers
D. GI bleeding
E. Colitis

Q2.4 In Zollinger–Ellison syndrome:

A. Gastrinomas are commonest in the tail of the pancreas
B. 50% or more gastrinomas are malignant
C. Gastrinomas metastatic to the lymph nodes have a worse prognosis than those to the liver
D. Vitamin B12 is malabsorbed due to lack of intrinsic factor
E. Gastric rugal hypertrophy may occur

Q2.5   Gastric cancer is very common in:

A. The Confederation of Independent States
B. The United States of America
C. Japan
D. Southern Italy
E. West Africa

Q2.6   In actively bleeding duodenal ulcers options in therapy include:

A. Laser treatment
B. Adrenaline injection
C. Heater probe coagulation
D. Open surgery
E. Transfusion

Q2.7   A middle-aged woman is admitted with Hb 3.8 g/dl, MCV 64 fl. Previous investigation for severe iron deficiency anaemia had shown only antral gastritis and sigmoid diverticulosis. She had been transfused blood one year before and numerous courses of iron supplements over the previous five years. Gastroscopy was repeated and showed antral gastritis in the form of streaks appearing to converge on the pylorus. Biopsies showed dilated ectatic vessels. Her anaemia is likely to be due to:

A. Sigmoid diverticulosis
B. Hereditary haemorrhagic telangiectasia
C. Water-melon stomach
D. Hp associated gastritis
E. None of these

Q2.8   *Helicobacter pylori*:

A. Efficacy of eradication is best confirmed by serology
B. Result of ^{13}C urea breath test can be affected by medical therapy
C. Culture and sensitivity is now fairly widely available in hospital practice
D. PCR (polymerase chain reaction) techniques are not commonly used in clinical practice
E. CLO-test is more sensitive and specific than ^{13}C urea breath test

Q2.9   In management of benign gastric ulcer treatment with the following are used:

A. Felodipine
B. Famotidine
C. Nimodipine
D. Nizatidine
E. Tinidazole

Q2.10 Peak acid output is a technique useful in assessment of:

A. Success of vagotomy
B. Diagnosis of peptic ulcer
C. Presence of pernicious anaemia
D. Analysis of dyspepsia
E. Presence of endocrine tumours

Q2.11 *Helicobacter pylori* infection is associated with:

A. Barrett's oesophagus
B. Antral gastritis
C. Peptic ulcer
D. Carcinoid syndrome
E. Gastric lymphoma

Q2.12 A 61-year-old woman with a history of vagotomy and pyloroplasty 30 years before for peptic ulcer disease develops right-sided abdominal aching and backache which is constant for 5 months. She is more likely than ordinary people to have:

A. Gastrinoma
B. Hypercalcaemia
C. Gallstones
D. Chronic pancreatitis
E. Porphyria

Q2.13 In patients with atrophic gastritis:

A. Pernicious anaemia is common
B. A gastric ulcer is often present
C. There is an increased incidence of gastric cancer
D. The Schilling test is normal
E. 5% of patients secrete acid in response to pentagastrin

Q2.14 In patients admitted to hospital with acute upper gastro-intestinal haemorrhage:

A. Some form of chronic peptic ulcer is the commonest diagnosis
B. Gastric ulcer is commoner than duodenal ulcer
C. Mallory–Weiss syndrome is exceedingly rare
D. Only about 50% of patients known to have oesophageal varices are actually bleeding from them
E. With the widespread use of endoscopy in the last few years the mortality rate has fallen dramatically

Q2.15 Which of the following external signs have been described in association with gastric neoplasms:

A. Weight loss
B. Lymph node metastasis in the neck
C. Necrobiosis lipoidica
D. Carcinoid flush
E. Acanthosis nigricans

Q2.16 *Helicobacter pylori*:

A. Causes gastric lymphoma
B. Colonises normal duodenal mucosa
C. Is an anaerobic organism
D. Leads to the formation of neutralising antibodies
E. Can be eradicated from the stomach by treatment with antibiotics alone

Q2.17 Proton pump inhibitor drugs:

A. Reduce serum gastrin concentrations
B. Bind to hydrogen/potassium ATPase on the parietal cell
C. May interfere with the metabolism of warfarin
D. Cause regression of Barrett's oesophagus
E. Increase susceptibility to enteric infection with salmonella

Q2.18 Gastrin:

A. Is secreted by G cells in the gastric fundus
B. Stimulates water and electrolyte secretion from the stomach
C. Inhibits electrolyte absorption in the jejunum
D. Is found in abnormally high levels in the serum of patients with pernicious anaemia
E. May be secreted by pancreatic tumours resulting in the Verner–Morrison syndrome

Q2.19 The following statements about endoscopy are correct:

A. It is often performed without sedation
B. Disinfection is now exclusively with glutaraldehyde
C. Stones in the gallbladder may be extracted at ERCP
D. Some gastric polyps may safely be left *in situ*
E. PEG (percutaneous endoscopic gastrostomy) tube is a good treatment for intractable tight oesophageal stricture

Q2.20 Gastric carcinoma:

A. Has a 5-year survival in best UK centres of around 80%
B. Is linked epidemiologically with *H. pylori* infection
C. If detected very early, may have 5-year survival of 95%
D. Can heal with acid suppressant therapy
E. Is more common in blood group A

Q2.21 Gastric *Helicobacter pylori* infection can be identified by the following techniques:

A. Haemotoxylin and eosin
B. Giemsa
C. Toluidine blue
D. Electron microscopy
E. Warthin Starry

Q2.22 Osler–Weber–Rendu syndrome (hereditary haemorrhagic telangiectasia) (HHT):

A. Presents with GI blood loss from the second decade onwards
B. May be associated with pulmonary and neurological disease
C. Is caused by mutations within the TGF-β receptor gene
D. Can have recurrent transfusion requirements even in oestrogen therapy
E. May be cured by surgery

Q2.23 When testing for the presence of *Helicobacter pylori*:

A. False positives are obtained if a proton pump inhibitor has been given in the preceding week
B. Serology tests are used to demonstrate persistent active infection
C. A silver stain is usually used to detect it histologically
D. The CLO-test should be read at one hour
E. Serology rapidly changes when *H. pylori* has been successfully treated

Q2.24 In a patient presenting with upper gastrointestinal bleeding:

A. Mortality increases with age
B. IV H2 receptor antagonists are useful in preventing rebleeding
C. Immediate endoscopy is required
D. Active bleeding at endoscopy is an indication for surgery
E. A clean ulcer base at endoscopy is rarely associated with further bleeding

Q2.25 The following are effective in reducing the risk of bleeding when varices are known to be present:

A. Isosorbide mononitrate
B. Propranolol
C. Ascitic tap
D. Bisoprolol
E. Liver transplant

Q2.26 How many drugs are necessary for reliable eradication of *Helicobacter pylori*?

A. 1
B. 2
C. 3
D. 4
E. 5

Q2.27 In spontaneous bleeding peptic ulcer:

A. High dose proton pump inhibitor therapy can reduce bleeding
B. Injection sclerotherapy is superior to adrenaline injection
C. Early surgery is not usually required
D. *Helicobacter pylori* eradication therapy is useful
E. Mortality is very low under 65 years

Q2.28 A 65-year-old woman presents with anaemia, low serum folate but normal mean corpuscular volume (MCV). Three occult blood tests in the stool are positive:

A. Gastroscopy and small bowel biopsy are indicated
B. Sigmoidoscopy and colonoscopy or barium enema will probably be necessary
C. Diverticular disease may be the only finding
D. Carcinoma of the colon is not likely
E. In-patient investigation is essential

Q2.29 Gastric cancer:

A. Is usually curable by radical surgery
B. Is defined as early when limited to mucosa and sub-mucosa
C. Is associated with *Helicobacter pylori*
D. May be caused by gastric surgery
E. Is associated with coeliac disease

Q2.30 In patients admitted with upper gastrointestinal haemorrhage, rebleeding is likely if endoscopy reveals:

A. Reflux oesophagitis
B. A peptic ulcer with a clean white base
C. A peptic ulcer with a visible vessel
D. Oesophageal varices
E. A Mallory–Weiss tear

Q2.31 A 70-year-old lady presents with anorexia, a feeling of early satiety and weight loss. Examination is normal, except she is pale. The laboratory report that she has a micro-angiopathic haemolytic anaemia. Likely diagnoses include:

A. Ulcerative colitis with malignant change in the colon
B. Haemochromatosis with cirrhosis
C. Crohn's disease of the duodenum
D. Linitis plastica
E. Polycystic kidneys

Q2.32 *Helicobacter pylori* eradication therapy has been associated with:

A. A reduction in gastric carcinoma incidence
B. Curative therapy for gastric MALT lymphoma
C. Increased gastro-oesophageal reflux
D. Decreased rates of eradication if there has been pretreatment with proton pump inhibitors (PPI)
E. Development of significant drops in intragastric pH

Q2.33 An 80-year-old lady with a known hiatus hernia, is admitted with a sudden onset of dysphagia, inability to vomit and shock. Intravenous fluids, analgesia and oxygen are administered. What procedures might be helpful next:

A. Chest x-ray
B. CT scan of thorax and abdomen
C. Mesenteric angiogram
D. Passage of a nasogastric tube
E. Gastroscopy

Q2.34 The following features are predictors of rebleeding in peptic ulcers presenting with haemorrhage:

A. Use of NSAIDs (non-steroidal anti-inflammatory drugs)
B. Smoking
C. Age > 60
D. A visible vessel in the base of an ulcer
E. The presence of melaena

Q2.35 Gastric ulcer:

A. Relapses frequently even when *Helicobacter pylori* is eradicated
B. Is associated with *Helicobacter* in > 90% of those cases in which NSAIDs are not implicated
C. Usually presents by the age of 50
D. Is less likely to be malignant if found on the greater curve than the lesser
E. Usually occurs in patients with a high basal acid secretion

Q2.36 A 38-year-old woman was shown to have a duodenal ulcer at endoscopy. After therapy with lansoprazole, amoxycillin and metronidazole she was cured of dyspepsia for two years. A carbon-14 urea breath test was negative after treatment. She then developed a relapse of dyspepsia with heartburn:

A. Recrudescence of *H. pylori* and peptic ulcer is likely
B. Symptomatic therapy is all that is needed
C. Development of gastro-oesophageal reflux disease is likely
D. Repeat endoscopy with urease test is required
E. Treatment with antacids will not obscure the diagnosis

Q2.37 Gastric cancer:

A. Is increasing in incidence in the Western World
B. Is the second commonest fatal cancer in the world
C. Is weakly associated with *Helicobacter*
D. Is associated with low intake of antioxidant vitamins in the diet
E. Is associated with a steadily improving prognosis over the last 10 years

Q2.38 These anti-platelet drugs frequently cause gastrointestinal (GI) bleeding:

A. Ticlopidine
B. Dipyridamole
C. Meloxicam
D. Aspirin
E. Clopidogrel

Q2.39 Which of the following drugs reduce gastric acid secretion:

A. Omeprazole
B. Ranitidine
C. Misoprostol
D. Pirenzepine
E. Sucralfate

2. Answers

A2.1
A. True
B. False
C. False
D. True
E. False

Spontaneous duodenal ulcer is almost always linked with *Helicobacter pylori* infection. Many older regimes with low efficacy cannot be trusted to have worked. If the patient has *H. pylori* antibodies in the serum this may only mean past infection, though they would also be present in current disease. Urea breath testing accurately reflects current infection if the patient has not recently been on proton pump inhibitor, bismuth or antibiotic therapy. The fatality rate is vanishingly small under the age of 60 years in uncomplicated duodenal ulcer.

A2.2
A. True
B. True
C. True
D. True
E. True

Haemorrhage is much the commonest. Gastric outflow obstruction and perforation are much less frequently seen. Ulcers may penetrate into the pancreas giving acute inflammation. Peptic ulcer disease may occasionally obstruct the ampulla leading to obstructive jaundice.

A2.3
A. False
B. False
C. True
D. True
E. True

These drugs cause, prevent healing of, and precipitate bleeding from peptic ulcers. They are not associated with oesophageal disease. They will worsen symptoms in inflammatory bowel disease.

A2.4

A. False
B. True
C. False
D. False
E. True

In Zollinger–Ellison syndrome pancreatic gastrinomas commonly occur in the head of the pancreas, but as many as two thirds of patients may have extra-pancreatic gastrinomas. One half to two thirds of gastrinomas are malignant. Hepatic metastasis (but not lymph node involvement) is associated with a poor prognosis. Steatorrhoea and vitamin B12 malabsorption may occur – low intestinal pH interferes with vitamin B12 absorption, though intrinsic factor secretion is normal. Gastric rugal hypertrophy similar to Menetrier's disease may occur.

A2.5

A. True
B. False
C. True
D. False
E. False

Gastric carcinoma prevalence is moderate and falling in the USA, Western Europe and the Antipodes. Both Japan and the countries of the old communist bloc have very high rates.

A2.6

A. True
B. True
C. True
D. True
E. True

All of these can be used. Appropriate resuscitation with transfusion, endoscopy to identify the problem, and adrenaline injection are baseline procedures. The laser and heater probe are probably equivalent to adrenaline injection but not superior. Surgery is generally reserved for repeat or refractory bleeding.

A2.7
A. False
B. False
C. True
D. False
E. False

Water-melon stomach is an uncommon but well recognised cause of severe iron deficiency anaemia, more common in women. If anaemia persists despite continuing oral iron supplements treatment options consist of endoscopic therapy, corticosteroids, oestrogen/progesterone preparations and antrectomy.

A2.8
A. False
B. True
C. False
D. True
E. False

A2.9
A. False
B. True
C. False
D. True
E. True

Famotidine and nizatidine are alternative H2 receptor antagonist gastric acid anti-secretory drugs. Tinidazole is used in combinations against *H. pylori*. Felodipine and nimodipine are calcium channel blocking agents used in vascular diseases.

A2.10
A. True
B. False
C. True
D. False
E. True

After vagotomy peak acid output falls. Studies before and after surgery are needed. In pernicious anaemia there is achlorhydria, but this can occur in other conditions too. Gastrinoma will lead to a raised basal acid output which is the same as the peak acid output, which itself is either high or at the upper end of the normal range.

A2.11
A. False
B. True
C. True
D. False
E. True

Helicobacter pylori is not linked with gastro-oesophageal reflux disease: indeed eradication of infection may precipitate this problem. *H. pylori* does cause peptic ulcers and gastric lymphomas (MALToma). It has also been linked with gastric carcinoma and ischaemic heart disease.

A2.12
A. False
B. False
C. True
D. True
E. False

If peptic ulcer disease is caused by metabolic problems such as raised gastrin or calcium it would not lie dormant for decades after vagotomy. This operation does alter gallbladder motility so that gallstone prevalence is increased. Patients who come to gastric surgery are more likely than the rest of the population to be smokers and heavy alcohol users, so pancreatitis should be considered.

A2.13
A. True
B. False
C. True
D. False
E. False

A2.14
A. True
B. False
C. False
D. True
E. False

A2.15
A. True
B. True
C. False
D. True
E. True

A2.16
A. True
B. False
C. True
D. False
E. True

A2.17
A. False
B. True
C. True
D. False
E. True

A2.18
A. False
B. True
C. True
D. True
E. False

Gastrin is mainly produced and secreted by the G cells in the gastric antrum. Its many actions include stimulation of gastric acid, water and electrolyte secretion, inhibition of water and electrolyte absorption in the lower small intestine, promotion of gut motility and trophic effects on the gastric mucosa. Abnormally high levels may be found in the blood of patients with pernicious anaemia. Some pancreatic tumours secrete gastrin resulting in excessive acid secretion and the symptoms of Zollinger–Ellison syndrome. The excessive secretion of vasoactive intestinal polypeptide (VIP) causes the severe diarrhoea and electrolyte disturbances seen in Verner–Morrison syndrome.

A2.19
A. True
B. True
C. False
D. True
E. False

A2.20
A. False
B. True
C. True
D. True
E. True

A2.21
A. True
B. True
C. True
D. True
E. True

A2.22
A. False
B. True
C. True
D. True
E. False

In HHT affected families have been found to have mutations in the TGF-β gene and usually develop epistaxis in the second decade and develop GI bleeding from the fifth decade onwards. HHT is associated with both pulmonary and CNS arteriovenous malformations which can be complicated by pulmonary shunting and cerebrovascular accidents. Oestrogens remain the only medical therapy shown to decrease transfusion requirements. Surgery is not curative as further telangiectatic lesions develop.

A2.23
A. False
B. False
C. False
D. False
E. False

The gold standard for detecting *H. pylori* is culture but this is technically difficult and takes some time. The modified Giemsa stain is used for histological diagnosis. The CLO-test should be read finally at 24 hours, to avoid false negatives.

A2.24
A. **True**
B. **False**
C. **False**
D. **False**
E. **True**

In patients presenting with upper GI bleeding endoscopy should be performed after initial resuscitation. Failure to control active bleeding at endoscopy would be an indication for surgery. There is no evidence that IV H2 receptor antagonists reduce morbidity and mortality. Endoscopic findings of adherent clot, non-bleeding visible vessel or active bleeding of an ulcer carry an increased risk of rebleeding.

A2.25
A. **True**
B. **True**
C. **False**
D. **False**
E. **True**

Nitrates combined with a non-cardioselective beta-blocker are said to be as effective as variceal injection sclerotherapy for reducing the rate of rebleeding from varices. Bisoprolol is too cardioselective to be effective.

A2.26
A. **False**
B. **True**
C. **True**
D. **True**
E. **False**

No one drug is reliable; five are unnecessary. Regimes with clarithromycin plus ranitidine bismuth citrate have been effective if costly. Generally, however, three to four drugs including a proton pump inhibitor and at least two antibiotics give the best results. Unless 90%+ success rates can be demonstrated, therapy cannot nowadays be recommended.

A2.27
A. True
B. False
C. True
D. True
E. True

The chance of younger patients dying of bleeding peptic ulcer is small: the older patients are often victims of concomitant disease rather than gastrointestinal haemorrhage itself. Though standard doses of anti-acid therapy have been disappointing, the use of e.g. omeprazole 40 mg b.d. for 5 days seems to be beneficial. Adrenaline injection into ulcer bases is known to be effective, but it is unclear whether any other additional agents improve results. Bleeding usually settles spontaneously and radical cure with anti-*Helicobacter pylori* therapy will prevent recurrence.

A2.28
A. True
B. True
C. True
D. False
E. False

Bleeding peptic ulcer, carcinoma of the stomach and coeliac disease are all possible and need to be excluded. Multiple pathology is quite possible, and large bowel investigations are necessary. Diverticular disease is common, but does not exclude carcinoma of the large bowel or inflammatory bowel disease which are also common. Most of these patients should be investigated as out-patients.

A2.29
A. False
B. True
C. True
D. True
E. False

The majority of cases are not curable by surgery at the time of diagnosis, unless the cancer is early. Even when the cancer is early local lymph nodes may be involved. 70% of gastric cancer patients have *Helicobacter pylori*. Partial gastrectomy is a risk factor for gastric cancer with a five-fold increase in risk after 20 years. Coeliac disease is associated with small intestinal lymphomas and adenocarcinomas along with oesophageal cancer but not gastric cancer.

A2.30
A. False
B. False
C. True
D. True
E. False

Reflux oesophagitis is an unusual cause of severe GI bleeding and an even rarer cause of rebleeding. Peptic ulcers with a clean white base rebleed rarely but when a visible vessel is present rebleeding occurs in 50%. Oesophageal varices commonly rebleed, but although Mallory–Weiss tears do so occasionally, it is uncommon.

A2.31
A. False
B. False
C. False
D. True
E. False

Micro-angiopathic haemolytic anaemia is frequently associated with carcinomatosis, and a common site is carcinoma of the stomach. The diagnosis of this lady's linitis plastica was made by the haematologist prior to endoscopy.

A2.32
A. False
B. True
C. True
D. False
E. True

Helicobacter pylori eradication is curative in up to 74% of low grade MALT lymphomas. Despite the strong epidemiological evidence suggesting a role for *H. pylori* in gastric carcinogenesis, there is no evidence yet that eradication therapy leads to a decrease in gastric cancer incidence. Pre-treatment with PPIs has not been found to affect eradication rates. Successful eradication leads to a drop in gastric pH and increased symptoms of GORD.

A2.33
A. True
B. False
C. False
D. False
E. True

This is a characteristic picture of acute gastric volvulus occurring as a complication of a para-oesophageal ('rolling') hiatus hernia. The whole stomach revolves on its axis producing an obstruction at both ends of the stomach.

A chest x-ray will show dilatation of the fundus and pylorus with fluid levels in both areas. A CT scan will not alter management. Mesenteric angiography can be diagnostic, but in most cases will merely delay effective treatment which is surgery. Attempted passage of a naso-gastric tube will be unsuccessful. Endoscopic decompression has been reported, and in very experienced hands may be helpful.

A2.34
A. False
B. False
C. False
D. True
E. False

A2.35
A. False
B. True
C. False
D. False
E. False

Gastric ulcer, when it is not associated with NSAIDs, occurs in stomachs with a pangastritis, and in an older age group (> 50 years). The often quoted figure of 70% *Helicobacter* positivity in gastric ulcer does not take account of those caused by NSAIDs, nor of gastric atrophy which is often present and makes the organisms scarce, nor of the declining serological response which occurs with age and scarcity of the organisms and gives rise to false negatives. Studies on stored sera confirm a similar infection rate (more than 90%) for gastric ulcer as for duodenal ulcer. The pangastritis accounts for the low acid output usually found in these patients.

A2.36
A. False
B. False
C. True
D. True
E. True

The most likely explanation is gastro-oesophageal reflux disease, which sometimes appears to be precipitated by successful anti-*Helicobacter pylori* therapy. However, it is important to exclude recurrent peptic ulcer disease and gastroscopy with urease testing will do this. Prior to investigation it is best to avoid ulcer healing treatment and antibiotics which will alter the result. At this length of time the serum *H. pylori* ELISA test should be negative after successful therapy, though this sero-conversion takes 6–12 months after treatment.

A2.37
A. False
B. True
C. False
D. True
E. False
The incidence of gastric cancer has been steadily declining for much of this century in developed societies, such that in the UK the annual incidence has dropped from 12 000 to c. 8000 over the last decade. Nevertheless world-wide it remains a very common cancer. The prognosis has altered little with poor five-year survival rates being the norm. Although studies have shown improved survival with early detection, most cancers continue to present late. The association with *Helicobacter pylori* is strong with, for instance, the Eurogast study showing an increased risk of two- to six-fold for *Helicobacter* infected populations. Poor intake of vitamin C and high exposure of the gastric mucosa to nitrates and nitrosamines are also risk factors.

A2.38
A. False
B. False
C. False
D. True
E. False
GI bleeding is doubled by aspirin 75 mg daily, trebled by 150 mg daily, quadrupled by 300 mg daily and increased six-fold by 1200 mg daily. It is the most useful anti-platelet drug, but the lowest effective dose should always be used.

Meloxicam is a non-steroidal anti-inflammatory drug with cyclo-oxygenase-2 inhibitory activity and is claimed to have a low incidence of GI side-effects, but does not have anti-platelet activity.

A2.39
A. True
B. True
C. True
D. True
E. False

Omeprazole blocks the gastric H^+K^+-ATPase, whereas ranitidine and pirenzepine block the receptors on the gastric parietal cell. Misoprostol and sucralfate have 'cytoprotective' properties, and misoprostol also has an anti-secretory property which accounts for some of its ulcer healing action.

3. Absorption and the Intestine

Q3.1 A 27-year-old woman had two resections for terminal ileal Crohn's disease 5 years and 4 months before. She attended clinic complaining of hypomenorrhoea, abdominal aching, and pains in both anterior thighs. There was no nausea, altered bowel habit or weight loss. On examination there was a tender 5 × 15 cm mass in the right iliac fossa. Gait was normal.

A. White cell scan would be useful
B. Local sepsis is more likely than recurrent Crohn's disease
C. An iliopsoas abscess needs to be excluded
D. Treatment with steroids is likely to be required
E. Metronidazole may be used

Q3.2 Gastrointestinal tract lymphoma:

A. Is a rare site of non-nodal involvement
B. Is almost exclusively non-Hodgkin's lymphoma
C. May complicate *H. pylori* infection
D. Frequently involves the terminal ileum
E. Of the MALT type involving the stomach is characteristically disseminated at the time of diagnosis

Q3.3 Coeliac disease is characteristically associated with deficiency of:

A. Vitamin A
B. Vitamin B
C. Vitamin C
D. Vitamin D
E. Vitamin E

Q3.4 Diseases which normally require anti-microbial treatment are:

A. Oesophageal candida
B. Peptic ulcers
C. Whipple's disease
D. Gastroenteritis
E. Shigella dysentery

Q3.5   A 28-year-old man with a history of terminal ileal resection 7 years before for Crohn's disease develops new right-sided abdominal pain. Tests which would help in diagnosis include:

A. SeHCAT scanning for bile acid absorption
B. White blood cell scan
C. Schilling test
D. Flexible sigmoidoscopy
E. Barium meal

Q3.6   A 35-year-old insulin dependent diabetic female presents with chronic diarrhoea:

A. A large stool osmotic gap is consistent with sorbitol induced diarrhoea
B. A positive anti-endomysial antibody test would have no diagnostic value
C. Bacterial overgrowth is a common aetiology
D. Clonidine therapy may be useful in increasing reabsorption of fluid
E. Faecal fat may be elevated

Q3.7   A 25-year-old lady with steroid-dependent Crohn's disease is being considered for immunosuppressive therapy. Toxicity related to azathioprine treatment of Crohn's disease:

A. Can be ameliorated by concurrent administration of allopurinol
B. May be genetically determined
C. Contra-indicates its use in pregnancy
D. Includes frequent incidence of non-Hodgkin's lymphoma
E. Prevents administration of this drug in 50% of the patients

Q3.8   Intestinal bacterial overgrowth can occur in the following conditions:

A. Following Billroth 2 gastrectomy
B. Hypothyroidism
C. Diverticular disease of the colon
D. Ulcerative colitis
E. Diabetes mellitus

Q3.9   Jejunoileal bypass (JIB) for morbid obesity:

A. Leads to inadequate weight loss
B. Has been superseded by other gastrointestinal operations
C. Facilitates a reduction in food intake
D. Can be complicated by serious electrolyte disturbances
E. Is well tolerated by some patients

Q3.10 The following conditions cause a secretory diarrhoea:

A. Cholera
B. *E. coli* O157 food poisoning
C. Disaccharidase deficiency
D. Lactulose treatment
E. Irritable bowel syndrome

Q3.11 A 75-year-old arteriopath is rushed to hospital with a history of severe acute abdominal pain, vomiting and diarrhoea. On admission he is hypotensive and pale with abdominal distention but normal bowel sounds. Tests likely to give a diagnosis are:

A. Plain x-ray of abdomen
B. Abdominal ultrasound
C. Mesenteric angiography
D. Urgent barium enema
E. Small bowel follow-through examination

Q3.12 In patients with coeliac disease:

A. Oral aphthous ulcers are likely to improve on a gluten-free diet
B. The serum is likely to contain reticulin antibodies, particularly in children
C. Small intestinal lymphoma can be a complication even in subjects who have been on a gluten-free diet for many years
D. The small bowel histology is specific to the diagnosis
E. The symptoms may be improved by omitting milk products from the diet

Q3.13 Which of the following conditions may complicate Crohn's disease:

A. Sacro-iliitis
B. Macroglossia resulting from amyloidosis
C. Distal interphalangeal joint polyarthritis
D. Increased incidence of cholesterol gallstones
E. Increased incidence of oxalate renal stones

Q3.14 Coeliac disease:

A. Can occur in patients over 60 years old
B. Has a familial incidence
C. Frequently presents as anaemia
D. Is associated with an increased incidence of small intestinal lymphoma
E. Always responds to withdrawal of gluten from the diet

Q3.15 A 52-year-old man presented with diarrhoea and flushing episodes. Urinary 5-HIAA was elevated. In carcinoid tumours:

A. High urinary 5-HIAA concentrations indicate a poor prognosis
B. Somatostatin receptors are not expressed
C. The carcinoid syndrome occurs more commonly with hindgut tumours than foregut tumours
D. Rectum is the commonest site of hindgut involvement
E. Liver metastasis indicates a poor 5-year survival of 5% or less

Q3.16 Often associated with Crohn's disease are:

A. Familial history
B. Finger clubbing
C. Fistula in ano
D. Pneumaturia
E. Hypercalcaemia

Q3.17 Nitric oxide:

A. Is a neurotransmitter in the CNS
B. Is a neurotransmitter in the myenteric plexus
C. Is an endorphin
D. Given intravenously, can help maintain blood pressure in shocked patients
E. Is produced in most tissues by metabolism of lysine

Q3.18 Features of Whipple's disease include:

A. Weight loss
B. Arthralgia
C. Diarrhoea
D. Yellow nails
E. Skin pigmentation

Q3.19 Irritable bowel syndrome (IBS):

A. May occur as a consequence of enteric infection
B. Is more frequent in women than men
C. Is usually associated with chronic proctitis on rectal biopsy
D. Partially responds to therapy with serotonin ($5HT_1$) antagonists
E. Is almost always associated with reduced thresholds of visceral sensation in the rectum

Q3.20 A 42-year-old man with rheumatoid arthritis presented with recurrent abdominal pain and diarrhoea. The effect of non-steroidal anti-inflammatory drugs on the gut include:

A. Small intestinal strictures
B. Diaphragmatic septa in the mid small bowel
C. Protein losing enteropathy
D. Activation of inflammatory bowel disease
E. Decreased intestinal permeability

Q3.21 In coeliac disease the small bowel mucosa biopsy classically shows:

A. Flat mucosa
B. Increased mitotic index
C. Decreased intra-epithelial lymphocytes
D. Increased polymorphonuclears
E. Increased lymphocytes

Q3.22 In mesenteric angina:

A. The abdominal pain begins when the patient is eating
B. The presence of an abdominal bruit confirms the diagnosis
C. May lead to fatal acute intestinal infarction
D. Can be reliably diagnosed by Doppler ultrasound of the mesenteric vessels
D. May show diagnostic endoscopic appearances

Q3.23 Cholecystokinin:

A. Is a hormone produced by CCK cells within the small bowel in response to luminal fat
B. Relaxes the gallbladder and contracts the sphincter of Oddi
C. Stimulates appetite
D. Causes net fluid absorption from the colon
E. Stimulates bicarbonate secretion from pancreatic ductal cells

Q3.24 Intestinal lymphangiectasia:

A. Is a complication of non-Hodgkin's lymphoma
B. Is associated with a pleural effusion
C. Is treated by a high protein diet
D. Is diagnosed by endoscopic duodenal biopsies
E. Causes increased faecal fat output

Q3.25 Diarrhoea in AIDS patients:

A. Is usually due to opportunistic infection
B. Causes severe wasting and weight loss
C. Can be due to *Candida albicans*
D. Can be a source of HIV cross-infection
E. Leads to villous atrophy

Q3.26 Objective evidence to support a diagnosis of Crohn's disease relapse can be obtained from changes in:

A. C-reactive protein (CRP)
B. Platelets
C. Body mass index
D. Body temperature
E. Plasma globulins

Q3.27 A 6-month-old breast-fed baby has gastroenteritis. He looks approximately 5% dehydrated:

A. He should be rehydrated immediately with intravenous fluids
B. Mother should stop breast feeding for 24 hours
C. In the UK there is a 70% chance that he has a rotavirus infection
D. He should receive nothing but a glucose-electrolytes oral rehydration solution for 24 hours
E. The composition of the oral rehydration solution should be as recommended by the WHO and contain 90 mmol of sodium per litre

Q3.28 Which of these statements are true of tropical sprue:

A. In recent years the incidence in Britain has fallen considerably
B. Anaemia occurs as a result of iron and folic acid malabsorption
C. Peri-follicular haemorrhages and purpura may be associated with the disease
D. Radiological evidence of ileal involvement makes the diagnosis unlikely
E. A gluten-free diet should be advised

Q3.29 In coeliac disease:

A. There is an increased risk of Hodgkin's lymphoma
B. The incidence in Sweden is 3.5 per 1000 children and young adults
C. The incidence in Denmark is 0.1 per 1000 children and young adults
D. The risk of infertility is increased
E. The IgA anti-gliadin antibody assay is the most sensitive and specific screening test

Q3.30 In treatment of motility disorders:

A. Erythromycin is a good pro-kinetic agent
B. Domperidone crosses the blood–brain barrier
C. Cisapride acts at the level of the myenteric plexus
D. Cisapride has proved helpful in many irritable bowel patients
E. Nitrate relieves oesophageal spasm

Q3.31 Patients with coeliac disease:

A. Have undetectable anti-gliadin but persisting anti-endomysial antibodies after successful treatment
B. May benefit from pancreatic enzyme supplementation
C. Are at higher risk of microscopic colitis
D. Are more likely than a non-affected population to have Trisomy 21
E. May present with GI bleeding

Q3.32 The following breath tests can be used to diagnose bacterial overgrowth:

A. Hydrogen breath test with lactose
B. ^{14}C-glycocholate breath test
C. ^{14}C-triolein breath test
D. Hydrogen breath test with glucose
E. ^{14}C-urea breath test

Q3.33 Progressive systemic sclerosis may result in:

A. Small intestinal strictures
B. Bacterial colonisation
C. Intestinal pneumatosis
D. Achlorhydria
E. Oesophageal dysmotility which improves on steroid therapy

Q3.34 A balding middle-aged man with abnormal nails, complains of anorexia and weight loss. Gastroscopy shows multiple polyps. The likely diagnosis is:

A. Gardner's syndrome
B. Familial adenomatous polyposis syndrome
C. Ménétrièr's disease
D. Peutz–Jeghers' syndrome
E. Cronkite–Canada syndrome

Q3.35 A 30-year-old homosexual man has severe steroid responsive Crohn's colitis. Azathioprine has been give as a steroid sparing agent. If the steroids are stopped he relapses within a matter of weeks, and becomes severely ill and he has now been on steroids for 4 years. He doesn't wish for further surgery. Follow-up should include:

A. Regular eye checks
B. Blood count every 6 months
C. Thyroid function every 6 months
D. Bone densitometry
E. AIDS testing

Q3.36 A 36-year-old woman is admitted with a severe headache and neck stiffness. She has longstanding Crohn's disease, and is malnourished. The abdomen shows active peristalsis. Her arms are bruised. A cranial CT scan shows an intracerebral haemorrhage. What tests might lead to the underlying diagnosis:

A. Platelet count
B. Alpha 1 glycoprotein (oroso-mucoids)
C. Prothrombin time
D. MRI scan of abdomen
E. Carotid angiography

Q3.37 An elderly man presents with diarrhoea and swelling of his legs. Examination reveals steatorrhoea. His tests show a normal pancreas on ultrasound, a normal duodenal biopsy but an abnormal glycocholate breath test. What investigation might be helpful next:

A. Barium enema
B. Colonoscopy
C. Barium follow-through
D. Tubeless pancreatic tests
E. Anti-endomysial antibody

Q3.38 A 35-year-old woman with ileo-colonic Crohn's disease presents with difficulty walking. Examination reveals that she holds her right hip flexed and attempts to straighten it cause pain. What tests would lead quickest to the diagnosis:

A. Barium follow-through
B. Colonoscopy
C. CT scan of abdomen
D. X-ray of lumbar spine
E. Calcium level

Q3.39 In lactose intolerance:

A. The symptoms can be controlled by corticosteroids
B. A lactose-free diet is the treatment of choice
C. Jejunal biopsy histology is diagnostic
D. A rise in breath hydrogen by > 20 ppm in the first 2 hours after the ingestion of galactose indicates lactase deficiency
E. Yoghurt and cheeses may be tolerated in some cases

Q3.40 In coeliac disease:

A. Serum anti-gliadin antibodies remain the most sensitive and specific non-invasive tests for the condition
B. The chance of developing a lymphoma is unrelated to compliance with a gluten-free diet
C. Insulin-dependent diabetics are at increased risk of developing the condition
D. The chance of a patient with dermatitis herpetiformis also having small bowel biopsy evidence of coeliac disease is greater than 90%
E. HLA type B8 DR3 DQ2 is the commonest association in Northern Europe

Q3.41 In a pregnant patient with Crohn's disease who smokes:

A. Oral mesalazine therapy should be withdrawn
B. Oral corticosteroids are contra-indicated for disease relapse
C. Elemental diet is associated with foetal nutritional imbalance
D. The child has a one in six risk of developing inflammatory bowel disease
E. Continued smoking reduces risk of disease exacerbation

Q3.42 In a 34-year-old female presenting with a three-month history of diarrhoea, fatigue and low thoracic back pain, who has a normal full blood count, ESR, C-reactive protein, LFTs and TSH:

A. The symptoms are unlikely to be due to Crohn's disease
B. Chronic pancreatitis is excluded
C. Raised anti-gliadin and anti-endomysial antibodies are strongly pre-dictive of coeliac disease
D. If villous atrophy is found on duodenal biopsy, occult vitamin B12 deficiency is a common finding
E. The increased risk of gut lymphoma in coeliac disease is reduced by adherence to a gluten-free diet

Q3.43 Common presenting features in Crohn's disease include:

A. Pyrexia
B. Abdominal pain
C. Abdominal wall fistulas
D. Sacro-iliitis
E. Erythema nodosum

Q3.44 A small bowel biopsy showing sub-total villous atrophy in the adult is typically found in:

A. Coeliac disease
B. Lactase intolerance
C. Cystic fibrosis
D. Crohn's disease
E. Dermatitis herpetiformis

Q3.45 Following multiple resections of small bowel for recurrent Crohn's disease in a 26-year-old man, 180 cm of small bowel remain in the abdomen after his last operation:

A. There will be little absorption of secondary bile salts
B. Great adaptation will be possible if most of the bowel remaining is ileum
C. H2 blockade makes B12 deficiency more likely
D. Hyperuricaemia is more likely
E. Elemental diet will be necessary for nutrition to be maintained

Q3.46 A 28-year-old man presents with abdominal pain, loose stools and weight loss over 3 months. Colonoscopy is normal but small bowel barium x-ray demonstrates Crohn's disease of the mid ileum.

A. Crohn's disease is significantly associated with smoking
B. Sulphasalazine has a good chance of inducing remission in his case
C. Biopsy features of glandular destruction and crypt abscesses point to Crohn's disease rather than ulcerative colitis
D. Remission may be induced by restricting dietary intake to elemental feeding or total parenteral nutrition
E. Part of the cause of diarrhoea in this patient could be bile salt malabsorption

3. Answers

A3.1
A. True
B. False
C. True
D. True
E. True

Recurrent Crohn's disease proximal to the anastomosis is the most likely diagnosis, but local sepsis needs to be excluded before steroid therapy is given. A WBC scan and abdominal ultrasonography would both be helpful. Patients with iliopsoas abscess usually limp. Though metronidazole may be useful it is likely that steroid and immune suppressive treatment would be needed and repeat surgery would have to be considered.

A3.2
A. False
B. True
C. True
D. False
E. False

The gastrointestinal tract is a common site of non-nodal involvement by a non-Hodgkin's lymphoma. Though the terminal ileum has the highest concentration of mucosa associated lymphoid tissue (MALT), the stomach is the commonest site of involvement. *H. pylori* infection is associated with the formation of slow growing, localised gastric MALT lymphomas, which may be resectable, or may regress with *H. pylori* eradication.

A3.3
A. False
B. True
C. False
D. False
E. False

Though coeliac disease can cause steatorrhoea and deficiency of fat-soluble vitamins A, D and E, the most usual problem is folate deficiency leading to macrocytic anaemia. Iron deficiency also occurs.

A3.4
A. True
B. True
C. True
D. False
E. True

Topical and systemic anti-fungals will control thrush: antibiotics, steroid inhalers, and diabetes predispose to this condition. Eradication of *Helicobacter pylori* is a central part of spontaneous duodenal ulcer management. Whipple's disease is a chronic bacterial infection. Very prolonged treatment with tetracycline or co-trimoxazole is effective. Shigella infections are controlled by erythromycin or ciprofloxacin. Gastroenteritis is, however, normally self-limiting and antibiotics may worsen problems.

A3.5
A. False
B. True
C. False
D. False
E. False

After terminal ileal resection both bile acid and vitamin B12 absorption are likely to be affected, so SeHCAT and Schilling test will be abnormal anyway. By contrast, WBC scanning should indicate new active Crohn's disease lesions or sepsis. Barium meal and flexible sigmoidoscopy would not help with small bowel evaluation. Both small bowel enema and barium enema could be useful, however.

A3.6
A. True
B. False
C. False
D. True
E. True

Diabetic sweets often contain large amounts of sorbitol which may result in osmotic diarrhoea – the large osmotic gap would be accounted for by sorbitol which is unabsorbed. Coeliac disease is associated with diabetes and a positive anti-endomysial antibody in this patient would strongly suggest this diagnosis. Only a minority of patients will have documented bacterial overgrowth. Pancreatic insufficiency should be considered as a differential diagnosis of steatorrhoea associated with diabetes. GI adrenergic function is impaired in diabetic autonomic neuropathy and the α-2-adrenergic agonist clonidine has been successfully used in diabetic diarrhoea due to autonomic neuropathy by promoting fluid and electrolyte reabsorption and correcting motility disturbances. Octreotide therapy may also be useful.

A3.7

A. False
B. True
C. False
D. False
E. False

Allopurinol inhibits xanthine oxidase and delays the metabolism of azathioprine thus increasing toxicity. A genetically determined low level of activity of the enzyme thiopurine methyltransferase (TPMT) which partly inactivates 6-MP by methylation is responsible for myelotoxicity of azathioprine in a small number of patients. However, only 10% of patients fail to continue azathioprine due to side effects. Several normal pregnancies have occurred in patients on azathioprine and no teratogenicity has been reported. The decision to continue azathioprine in patients wishing to become pregnant needs to be discussed with the patient keeping in mind the consequences of disease relapse. A large cohort of patients followed up for a median of 15 years showed no increase in the incidence of cancers and lymphomas.

A3.8

A. True
B. True
C. False
D. False
E. True

Bacterial overgrowth occurs in small bowel diverticular disease, but not in colonic diverticular disease or in ulcerative colitis

A3.9

A. False
B. True
C. False
D. True
E. True

Jejunoileal bypass has been superseded by safer operations for morbid obesity. The early weight reduction was often good and is attributed to malabsorption because of the small bowel shunt. There is no restriction of food intake. About 50% of JIB patients developed serious late complications, e.g. electrolyte disturbances, liver disease, renal stones and arthritis. Surprisingly, the remainder achieved a reasonable weight without long-term problems. Thus it seems that some patients can tolerate a small bowel shunt better than others.

A3.10
A. True
B. True
C. False
D. False
E. False

Disaccharidase deficiency and lactulose treatment cause an osmotic diarrhoea. Irritable bowel syndrome is a motility problem. Cholera and *E. coli* infection cause a secretory diarrhoea mediated by cyclic AMP and adenylate cyclase.

A3.11
A. True
B. False
C. True
D. False
E. False

The history is suggestive of mesenteric infarction. Bowel sounds are often normal even in the face of severe infarction. Some patients have a surprisingly normal abdominal examination in spite of severe pain. Significant rectal bleeding would be suggestive of ischaemic colitis. Plain x-ray of abdomen will show evidence of air fluid levels and thick mucosal folds (thumb printing). An urgent mesenteric angiogram is mandatory before onset of irreversible necrosis and gangrene.

A3.12
A. True
B. True
C. True
D. False
E. True

A3.13
A. True
B. False
C. True
D. True
E. True

A3.14
A. True
B. True
C. True
D. True
E. False

A3.15
A. True
B. False
C. False
D. True
E. False

Urinary 5-HIAA correlates with the tumour load and prognosis. Carcinoid tumours express somatostatin receptors and hence can be imaged by radio-labelled octreotide scintigraphy. Rectum is the commonest site of hindgut involvement, but does not give rise to the carcinoid syndrome. Liver metastasis does not necessarily indicate a poor prognosis and 40%–60% 5-year survival is possible.

A3.16
A. True
B. True
C. True
D. True
E. False

A3.17
A. True
B. True
C. False
D. False
E. False

Nitric oxide, produced by metabolism of arginine, is a smooth muscle relaxant and produces vasodilation. It has a very short biological life, and can only be given via the inhalational route. It is produced in various tissues, including neurones, and is a neurotransmitter.

A3.18
A. True
B. True
C. True
D. False
E. True

Whipple's disease is a sub-acute illness caused by infection with *Tropheryma whippelii*, which can be identified by duodenal biopsy changes. It is characteristically a multisystem disease of middle-aged white males and requires prolonged antibiotic therapy: tetracycline plus folic acid up to a year has been used.

A3.19
A. True
B. True
C. False
D. False
E. False

Inflammation of the rectal mucosa precludes a sole diagnosis of irritable bowel syndrome. Heightened rectal sensation may be demonstrated in about half of individuals with irritable bowel syndrome seen by gastro-enterologists and possibly in a smaller proportion of IBS subjects in the community.

A3.20
A. True
B. True
C. True
D. True
E. False

NSAIDs set off a chain reaction of damage mediated by reactive oxygen metabolites resulting in disruption of the paracellular junction and in-creased intestinal permeability. NSAID associated strictures are commonly found in the mid small bowel, but may also occur in the ascending colon. The strictures have a range of appearances and include a characteristic diaphragmatic stricture. Iron deficiency anaemia, hypoproteinaemia owing to gut protein loss and intestinal obstruction may be presenting features. NSAIDs may activate subclinical inflammatory bowel disease within days of ingestion.

A3.21
A. True
B. True
C. False
D. False
E. True

A3.22
A. False
B. False
C. True
D. False
E. False

In mesenteric angina, the ischaemia caused by obstruction to the mesenteric vessels classically causes pain about 30 minutes after eating. Abdominal bruits are a common finding in patients with vascular disease and are of little diagnostic help. Doppler ultrasound may be helpful but is not sensitive enough to make the diagnosis without confirmation at mesenteric angiography. Colonoscopy may show appearances of ischaemic colitis but is not specific. In mesenteric angina, at least two of the three mesenteric vessels are occluded, and obstruction of the remaining patent vessel may cause fatal intestinal infarction.

A3.23
A. True
B. False
C. True
D. False
E. False

A3.24
A. True
B. True
C. False
D. True
E. False

A3.25
A. True
B. True
C. False
D. False
E. True

A3.26
A. True
B. True
C. True
D. True
E. True
As Crohn's is an inflammatory condition a range of systemic disturbances can be detected during a relapse.

A3.27
A. False
B. False
C. True
D. False
E. False

Rotavirus is the causative organism in approximately 70% of childhood gastroenteritis in the UK. Very few infants require intravenous rehydration and oral rehydration with a glucose-electrolyte solution should be tried first. Breast feeding should continue alongside oral rehydration therapy. Early refeeding shortens the illness and improves outcome, so starvation for 24 hours is no longer recommended. The WHO oral rehydration solution is designed for developing countries with different gut pathogens, where stool sodium loss may be very high. In the UK oral rehydration solution contains 30–60 mmol sodium per litre.

A3.28
A. False
B. True
C. True
D. False
E. False

A3.29
A. False
B. True
C. True
D. True
E. False

There is an increased incidence of non-Hodgkin's gut lymphomas in un-treated coeliac disease. Infertility, osteoporosis, and autoimmune diseases are also long-term risks. The great difference in incidence of coeliac disease in neighbouring Scandinavian countries with genetically similar populations may be explained by different infant feeding practices; Swedish infants receive much more gluten than their Danish counterparts. Endomysial antibody assay is the most specific and sensitive screening test for coeliac disease, but both this and the IgA anti-gliadin antibody test may be negative in selective IgA deficiency (in which there is an increased incidence of coeliac disease).

A3.30
A. True
B. False
C. True
D. True
E. True

A3.31
A. True
B. False
C. True
D. True
E. True
Coeliac disease is associated with an increased incidence of both colonic and pancreatic dysfunction. Serological tests, e.g. anti-gliadin, anti-reticulin and anti-endomysial antibodies decrease within months after commencing a gluten-free diet. Coeliac disease is found at high incidence in patients with Trisomy 21. Occult GI bleeding is commonly found in coeliac disease in addition to malabsorption of iron.

A3.32
A. False
B. True
C. False
D. True
E. False
Triolein is used to detect fat malabsorption, urea for *Helicobacter pylori* and lactose for lactase deficiency. Lactulose can, however, be used in a hydrogen breath test to detect bacterial overgrowth.

A3.33
A. False
B. True
C. True
D. False
E. False
Oesophageal involvement occurs in most patients with progressive systemic sclerosis. Reflux oesophagitis and oesophageal stricture may occur. Response to steroids is poor, but oesophageal dysmotility associated with mixed connective tissue disease appears to improve on steroid therapy. Typically the small bowel is dilated due to mural fibrosis. Pseudodiverticula, intestinal pneumatosis, intestinal pseudo-obstruction, volvulus and intussusception may occur. The hypomotility of the small bowel and jejunal diverticula cause stasis and bacterial colonisation leading to malabsorption. Gastric emptying of solids is delayed and gastric acid secretion is often increased, promoting oesophageal reflux mediated damage.

A3.34
A. False
B. False
C. False
D. False
E. True

Cronkite–Canada syndrome is a syndrome of generalised polyposis involving the stomach, small intestine and colon. Patients also have ectodermal features, including skin pigmentation, alopecia and dystrophic nails. It usually causes diarrhoea, severe malabsorption and protein using enteropathy and patients usually pursue a progressively downhill course.

A3.35
A. True
B. False
C. False
D. True
E. False

At present this man seems committed to long-term steroids. It is important to warn him of the risk of glaucoma and for him to have regular checks of his intra-ocular pressure. The British National Formulary recommends that the white count should be checked at least every 3 months after the initial 8 weeks. Bone densitometry should be considered – biphosphatase is now licensed as prophylaxis against steroid-induced osteoporosis.

A3.36
A. False
B. False
C. True
D. False
E. False

This lady has chronic malabsorption of vitamin K. Her prothrombin time was over 100 seconds and hence her bruising and spontaneous intracerebral haemorrhage. Intravenous vitamin K was administered and she fortunately settled without sequelae.

A3.37
A. False
B. False
C. True
D. False
E. False

The implication of his investigations is that he has steatorrhoea due to bacterial overgrowth, and a barium follow-through is the next investigation. It showed multiple duodenal diverticula. Treatment with tetracycline on a long-term basis led to complete resolution of his symptoms.

A3.38
A. False
B. False
C. True
D. False
E. False

The clinical picture is that of an ilio-psoas abscess. CT scanning is ideal for making this diagnosis and prompt surgery relieved her symptoms.

A3.39
A. False
B. True
C. False
D. False
E. True

Lactose intolerance is due to an absolute or partial lack of small bowel brush border lactase enzyme. About 5–15% of northern Europeans and Americans may be lactase deficient but in other parts of the world, i.e. Africa and Asia it may be as high as 75–100%. Avoidance of lactose-containing foods (predominantly milk) is the treatment, in areas where lactase deficiency is common milk is traditionally avoided but yoghurts and cheeses may be tolerated as they have low concentrations of lactose due to the effects of bacterial lactase. Light microscopy of the small bowel is normal. Specific enzyme analysis is required for absolute confirmation but intolerance is supported by the precipitation of symptoms after the ingestion of a lactose load and a rise in breath hydrogen > 20 ppm in the first 2 hours. A galactose test may be performed to eliminate a false positive result secondary to rapid intestinal transit.

A3.40
A. False
B. False
C. True
D. True
E. True

Anti-gliadin antibodies are associated with a proportion of false positives. Anti-endomysial antibodies which rely on antigen derived from monkey oesophagus show sensitivity and specificity approaching 100% in several studies. Anti-reticulin antibodies are specific but their sensitivity is less in adults than children. The chance of T-cell lymphoma is related to the length of time the disease has been present and to the cumulative antigen load encountered by the gut mucosa. Other GI malignancies such as oesophageal carcinoma and small bowel adenocarcinoma are over-represented but their aetiology is not understood. Other diseases associated with the B8 DR3 phenotype such as diabetes, thyroid disease and Addison's disease are found more frequently in coeliacs.

A3.41
A. False
B. False
C. False
D. True
E. False

Oral mesalazine is safe. Steroids have been used safely and extensively in pregnant patients with inflammatory bowel disease. There is no evidence to support the use of elemental diet. The risk in a first degree relative is increased to between 5% and 19%. Continued smoking increases the relapse rate and time to recurrence in Crohn's patients. Ex-smokers (and non-smokers) are at more risk of ulcerative colitis, where nicotine has been shown to have modest therapeutic efficacy.

A3.42
A. False
B. False
C. True
D. False
E. True

Crohn's disease may present with normal inflammatory markers, and back pain may result from associated ankylosing spondylitis. Whilst chronic pancreatitis may enter the differential diagnosis, it would be unusual in a young female, even in an alcoholic. Positive anti-gliadin antibodies alone are non-specific, but in combination with anti-endomysial antibodies and the clinical history, they suggest coeliac disease. Occult folate deficiency is not unusual, since folate is absorbed in the upper small intestine, where villous atrophy is most marked. Current evidence suggests that strict adherence to a gluten-free diet reduces the risk of certain associated malignancies; intestinal lymphoma, oesophagus, mouth and pharynx.

A3.43
A. True
B. True
C. False
D. False
E. True

Abdominal wall fistulas would only normally develop when Crohn's disease has been present for some time. Sacro-iliitis is an uncommon presenting feature in Crohn's disease.

A3.44
A. True
B. False
C. False
D. False
E. True

A3.45
A. True
B. False
C. False
D. True
E. False

The small bowel is 300–350 cm long and resection of 50% causes less absorption of nutrients and vitamins and may cause some wasting. Jejunum adapts better than ileum and symptoms of nutritional deficiency may improve after a time. Careful introduction of diet will be needed as hyperosmolar food will delay adaptation. Hypocalcaemia, arthritis, hyper-uricaemia and increased oxalic acid renal stones are all seen in this problem. Gastric hypersecretion may need treatment to prevent peptic ulceration. This treatment will not affect the co-factor for B12 absorption. The patient may need B12 to be given due to defective ileal absorption.

A3.46
A. True
B. False
C. False
D. True
E. True

Crohn's disease patients are more likely to be smokers than age and sex matched controls; the opposite applies to ulcerative colitis. Mesalazine is of uncertain value in Crohn's disease, especially in terms of inducing remission. Sulphasalazine is designed to release mesalazine in the colon, rather than the ileum. Granulomas are the pathognomonic histological feature of Crohn's disease but deep penetration of the inflammatory changes is also indicative. Exclusion of the normal diet from the gut can be an effective therapy in Crohn's disease but not in ulcerative colitis.

4. Large Bowel

Q4.1 A 20-year-old man presented with right lower quadrant pain and diarrhoea. Stool cultures grew *Yersinia enterocolitica* which:

A. May cause persistent ulceration of the terminal ileum
B. May cause enterocolic fistula
C. May present as 'acute appendicitis'
D. Is treated by penicillin
E. Is increased in incidence in haemochromatosis

Q4.2 A 69-year-old woman was admitted six weeks after a flu-like illness with a lower respiratory tract infection. She had received two courses of antibiotics and was given further alternative intravenous antibiotic therapy. Her fever remitted but then returned with diarrhoea and abdominal pain a week later:

A. Antibiotic therapy should be stopped
B. *Clostridium difficile* infection may be a problem
C. Sigmoidoscopy is always diagnostic of pseudomembranous colitis
D. Further treatment with metronidazole or vancomycin may be required
E. Fungal super-infection may be associated

Q4.3 Ischaemic colitis:

A. May occur in long distant runners
B. May complicate oral contraceptive pill usage
C. Usually affects the right side of the colon
D. Is characterised by haemosiderin-laden macrophages in the lamina propria
E. Is not associated with colonic dilatation

Q4.4 The requirement for colectomy in ulcerative colitis is nearest to:

A. 5%
B 15%
C. 50%
D. 75%
E. 100%

Q4.5   Collagenous colitis:

A. May be associated with rheumatoid arthritis
B. May improve after diversion ileostomy
C. Causes bloody diarrhoea indistinguishable from ulcerative colitis
D. Can be excluded if a rectal biopsy is normal
E. Is characterised by an increase in intra-epithelial lymphocytes

Q4.6   A 60-year-old man presents with rectal bleeding. He is found to have a soft, 1.5 cm diameter, pedunculated polyp in the rectum:

A. The lesion could be neoplastic
B. The lesion is likely to be benign
C. A full examination of the colon and rectum, either by colonoscopy or by double contrast barium enema, is essential
D. Total excision biopsy is indicated
E. Such lesions in the upper rectum should be treated by anterior resection

Q4.7   Appendicectomy:

A. Predisposes to ulcerative colitis
B. Is performed for normal appendices in 25% or more of cases
C. Is commoner in Crohn's disease
D. Is most frequent in children and young adults
E. Is commoner than in the nineteenth century

Q4.8   New treatments for acute severe ulcerative colitis include:

A. Azathioprine
B. Heparin
C. Cyclosporin
D. Lactose-free diet
E. Hemicolectomy

Q4.9   Drugs useful in colorectal carcinoma are:

A. Cyclosporin A
B. Ralitrexed
C. Folinic acid
D. Azathioprine
E. Fluorouracil

Q4.10 Inflammatory bowel disease:

A. Shows polygenic inheritance
B. Is an autosomal dominant disease
C. Is mainly environmentally determined
D. Shows greater concordance in blood relatives both for Crohn's disease and ulcerative colitis
E. Affects 1% or more of the population

Q4.11 Colonoscopy:

A. Is hazardous in patients with chronic obstructive airways disease
B. Requires prophylactic antibiotic therapy when undertaken in patients who have prosthetic heart valves
C. Is contra-indicated if ischaemic colitis is suspected
D. Can be used to visualise and biopsy the ileum
E. Is useful in the management of sigmoid volvulus

Q4.12 A 39-year-old man was given chemotherapy and cranial radiotherapy for acute leukaemia. He became severely neutropenic and developed a high fever, right lower quadrant abdominal pain and watery diarrhoea positive for occult blood. Reduced bowel sounds, colonic dilation on x-ray, and rigidity of the abdomen followed. The possible diagnoses are likely to include:

A. *Campylobacter* dysentery
B. Ulcerative colitis
C. *Clostridium difficile* infection
D. Giardiasis
E. Neutropenic enterocolitis

Q4.13 A 60-year-old obese man recently on a reducing diet with weight loss of 12 kg reports diarrhoea for years, with much slime and some bright blood mixed with the stool.

A. Flexible sigmoidoscopy is the logical first investigation
B. Barium enema is not required
C. Differential diagnoses include carcinoma, colitis and diverticular disease
D. If there is ulcerative colitis treatment will probably need to include surgery
E. Biopsy histology is important

Q4.14 In large bowel cancer adjuvant treatment after surgery usefully includes:

A. Radiotherapy
B. Fluorouracil and folinic acid
C. Fluorouracil and levamisole
D. High roughage diet
E. Stoma counselling

Q4.15 In the colonic epithelium:

A. Glutamine is the main energy source
B. Short chain fatty acids cannot be absorbed
C. Butyrate deficiency may lead to colitis
D. Bile acids promote water absorption
E. Short chain fatty acids promote cell proliferation

Q4.16 Carcinoma of the large bowel:

A. Is the commonest malignant tumour in Britain
B. Is familial
C. Can be predicted by genetic screening
D. Is usually caused by conditions such as ulcerative colitis or familial adenopolyposis of the colon
E. Is generally cured by surgery

Q4.17 A 19-year-old female with ulcerative colitis of the rectum and distal sigmoid colon only has intractable rectal bleeding:

A. Treatment with oral and topical mesalazine is beneficial
B. Systemic steroids may be required
C. The condition is self-limiting
D. Azathioprine may be effective
E. Local resection of the diseased bowel will cure the problem

Q4.18 A 65-year-old lady with advanced uterine carcinoma received 5 courses of radiation therapy to the pelvis. She presented complaining of diarrhoea. Radiation therapy to the pelvis may result in:

A. Rectovaginal fistula
B. Sigmoid colon stricture
C. Severe proctitis which may be cured by a defunctioning colostomy
D. Early damage to the vascular endothelium of the colon
E. Eosinophilic abscesses in the lamina propria

Q4.19 A middle-aged man has been treated for ulcerative colitis for several years. Which of the following are likely psychological concomitants:

A. Childlike dependence on the doctor
B. Depression
C. Anxiety
D. Denial of the severity of the illness
E. Hypochondriasis

Q4.20 A 35-year-old man presents with fever, malaise and bloody diarrhoea one year after a successful restorative procto-colectomy (RPC) with ileal pouch – anal anastomosis for ulcerative colitis:

A. He has a common complication of RPC
B. The likely cause is *Clostridium difficile* infection
C. Endoscopy and biopsy of the ileal pouch is indicated
D. He could have Crohn's disease rather than ulcerative colitis
E. Metronidazole therapy should be effective

Q4.21 Crohn's colitis:

A. Always requires total colectomy and ileo-anal pouch formation
B. May be complicated by sclerosing cholangitis
C. Can cause toxic megacolon
D. Predisposes to carcinoma of the colon
E. Responds to an elemental diet

Q4.22 Collagenous colitis:

A. Is common
B. Is associated with normal sigmoidoscopic appearances
C. Causes profuse watery diarrhoea
D. Is treated similarly to ulcerative colitis
E. Must be proved at biopsy

Q4.23 Which of the following symptoms are more commonly associated with Crohn's disease than with ulcerative colitis:

A. Bloody diarrhoea
B. Abdominal pain
C. Stricture formation
D. Peri-anal fissures and abscesses
E. Steatorrhoea

Q4.24 Which of the following investigations are indicated in a patient who develops recurrent episodes of severe abdominal pain and constipation:

A. Urinary urobilinogen content
B. Urinary delta-aminolaevulinate content
C. Kitchen tap water lead content
D. Urinary 5-hydroxytryptamine
E. Search for chylomicrons in the blood when fasting

Q4.25 In irritable bowel syndrome (IBS):

A. The site of the pain is of diagnostic value
B. The pain is typically worse after defecation
C. Weight loss is not a feature
D. Contrast radiology is required to confirm the diagnosis
E. There is an increase in the rectal mucosal vascular pattern

Q4.26 A 30-year-old man presents with severe peri-anal ulceration associated with a year's history of bloody diarrhoea. The cause may be:

A. Amoebiasis
B. Schistosomiasis
C. Tuberculosis
D. Gonorrhoea
E. Shigellosis

Q4.27 Solitary rectal ulcer syndrome is:

A. Excluded if more than one ulcer is present
B. Caused by digital trauma
C. A cause of rectal bleeding
D. Caused by a myenteric defect
E. Not diagnosable by histology

Q4.28 In inflammatory bowel disease (IBD):

A. Aminosalicylate (5-ASA) preparations are equally useful in both small and large bowel disease
B. Topical 5-ASA is less irritant to the rectum than foam steroid
C. Oral steroid is best given in divided daily doses
D. Both azathioprine and methotrexate are of proven value
E. Oral budesonide is licensed for both small and large bowel IBD

Q4.29 In familial adenomatous polyposis (FAP):

A. The presentation is usually in childhood
B. Small bowel polyps do not occur
C. There is a risk of death from desmoid tumours
D. We have the most common inherited genetic cause for colorectal cancer
E. Current practice is to perform prophylactic colectomy at around 20 years of age

Q4.30 Ischaemia of the large bowel:

A. May present with rectal bleeding
B. May present with abdominal colic
C. Involves the ascending colon most commonly
D. Causes deep rose-thorn ulcers in the acute phase
E. Is commonest in young Asians

Q4.31 Hair loss in ulcerative colitis is explained by:

A. Mesalazine therapy
B. Prednisolone therapy
C. Azathioprine therapy
D. Metronidazole therapy
E. Recovery from acute exacerbation

Q4.32 A 40-year-old man lost 10 kg in weight with diarrhoea but no blood loss over a six-week period. There was abdominal pain and hepatomegaly. On ultrasonography there were multiple filling defects in the liver. On flexible sigmoidoscopy there was a nodular circumferential infiltration of the recto-sigmoid with inflammation of the bowel above. Important differential diagnoses include:

A. Crohn's disease with associated liver disease
B. Ulcerative colitis with associated liver disease
C. Coeliac disease
D. Metastatic carcinoma of the rectum
E. AIDS

Q4.33 Features of a colorectal adenomatous polyp may include:

A. Dysplasia
B. Villous architecture
C. Increase in endocrine cells
D. Necrosis
E. Invasion of stalk

Q4.34 Colonoscopy:

A. Should be performed at three-yearly intervals on a 30-year-old patient whose parents both had colorectal carcinoma in their 40s
B. Needs to be repeated after 1–3 years to ensure a 'clean colon' after complete removal of a 1 cm tubulovillous adenoma at an initial colonoscopy
C. Is indicated in a patient with metaplastic sigmoid polyps
D. Is now recommended for all males over the age of 55 years, as a once-only screening test
E. Is needed in a patient with Crohn's total colitis which has been quiescent for 15 years

Q4.35 On histology of the appendix the following are not uncommon pathologies:

A. No significant abnormality
B. Fruit pips
C. Faecoliths
D. Threadworms
E. Diverticula

Q4.36 *Clostridium difficile* intestinal infection:

A. Occurs in 10% of the healthy population
B. Is always pathogenic
C. Increases to 45% after antibiotic treatment
D. Is frequent as a commensal in ulcerative colitis
E. Causes pseudomembranous colitis

Q4.37 Ulcerative colitis in a young woman:

A. Markedly reduces fertility
B. Greatly increases the chances of her child being stillborn
C. Usually deteriorates during pregnancy
D. Is most likely to relapse during the third trimester
E. Should not be treated with steroids during pregnancy because of the risk of fetal malformations

Q4.38 Colorectal cancer in the UK:

A. Is the third most common cause of death from malignancy
B. Accounts for about 19 000 deaths per year
C. Is amenable to 'curative' surgery in some cases
D. Rarely presents with distant metastases
E. Patients should be considered for adjuvant chemotherapy after 'curative' resection

Q4.39 A 15mm pedunculated recto-sigmoid polyp identified at sigmoidoscopy is biopsied and shows no evidence of dysplasia or malignancy:

A. No further action is required
B. Panproctocolectomy is the only safe option
C. Barium enema or colonoscopy is necessary
D. This is a rare finding
E. Excision by diathermy snare is likely to be the best option

Q4.40 Features of ulcerative colitis may include:

A. Sacro-iliitis
B. Aphthous ulceration in the mouth
C. Pyoderma gangrenosum
D. Erythema nodosum
E. Dermatitis herpetiformis

Q4.41 In investigation of suspected colonic disease in elderly patients:

A. Sigmoidoscopy is a logical first step
B. Barium enema without preparation is best
C. Diverticular disease is very common and may be incidental
D. Full colonoscopy yields more diagnoses than barium enema
E. CT scanning is a useful reserve test

Q4.42 Pneumatosis coli:

A. Affects large bowel only
B. Can be caused by diving
C. Can be diagnosed on barium enema
D. Responds to high flow oxygen
E. Usually spares the rectum

Q4.43 When treating inflammatory bowel disease:

A. 5-amino salicylic acid compounds treat relapses and maintain remission
B. Reversible interstitial nephritis is a side-effect of mesalazine
C. Azathioprine maintains remission in Crohn's disease
D. Azathioprine produces maximal response in 1–2 weeks
E. Cyclosporin maintains remission in ulcerative colitis

Q4.44 A 72-year-old lady reports diarrhoea since a bowel resection at age 32 for intestinal volvulus. What treatment might render her symptom free:

A. Steroids
B. Sulphasalazine
C. Pancreatic extract
D. Anti-oxidant therapy
E. Cholestyramine

Q4.45 A 30-year-old man with mild distal colitis presents with an exacerbation. Flexible sigmoidoscopy reveals multiple tiny ulcers extending to 20 cm from the anus and proximal to this the colon is normal. He has not lost weight. What treatment would you favour:

A. Intravenous steroids
B. Rectal steroids
C. Cyclosporin suppositories
D. Anti-oxidant therapy
E. Elemental diet

Q4.46 A 20-year-old female presents with a 9 month history of left iliac fossa pain, frequent bowel actions but no weight loss:

A. Abdominal bloating is pathognomic of an obstructing lesion leading to overflow diarrhoea
B. Associated with a variable stool consistency, urgency of defecation, relief of pain on defecation, is suggestive of the irritable bowel syndrome
C. Blood mixed with the stool indicates haemorrhoids
D. Gluten sensitive enteropathy is the most likely diagnosis
E. Anti-depressants are the treatment of first choice

Q4.47 In ulcerative colitis:

A. Using steroid enemas prevents the risk of systemic steroid side-effects
B. Liquid enemas only reach the sigmoid colon
C. Mesalazine enemas are effective in treating acute exacerbations
D. Regular colonoscopy has been demonstrated to reduce the mortality from bowel cancer
E. Acute renal failure may complicate the use of mesalazine

Q4.48 The lifetime risk of colonic cancer in a patient with one first-degree relative developing cancer of the colon aged greater than 45 is:

A. The same as in the general population
B. Ten times that of the general population
C. Three times that of the general population
D. Half that of the general population
E. Twice that of the general population

Q4.49 A 60-year-old farmer 10 years after abdomino-perineal resection of rectal carcinoma followed by radical radiotherapy developed a small bowel-cutaneous intestinal fistula:

A. The fistula is most likely to be from the distal jejunum
B. A sinogram is the first radiological investigation
C. Skin care will be a major therapeutic aim
D. Bowel rest is likely to be successful in closing the fistula
E. Histology of the resected bowel is likely to reveal endarteritis obliterans

Q4.50 A 72-year-old lady who had a 75% colectomy (and an ileo-colic anastomosis) for two synchronous colon cancers presented with diarrhoea and weight loss 4 years postoperatively. Diarrhoea had not been a problem following surgery:

A. Air in the colon on supine x-ray makes anastomotic recurrence likely
B. Two loops of slightly dilated jejunum signify partial small bowel obstruction
C. Normal carcino-embryonic antigen (CEA) levels and absence of a mass on computed tomography make recurrence unlikely
D. Diarrhoea is unlikely to be due to bacterial overgrowth
E. Laparotomy adesiolysis is likely to be helpful

Q4.51 A lady aged 82 years with known diverticular disease presented with 2 days vomiting, pyrexia, pain and tenderness in the left iliac fossa:

A. The most likely cause is large bowel obstruction
B. Early laparotomy may be indicated
C. Early passage of flatus means obstruction is not a problem
D. Urgent barium enema is needed to confirm the diagnosis
E. Intravenous cefuroxime and metronidazole is indicated

Q4.52 Complete rectal prolapse:

A. Is commonly associated with utero-vaginal prolapse in women
B. Is rare in nulliparous women
C. Is often associated with faecal incontinence
D. Sometimes needs to be distinguished from prolapsed haemorrhoids
E. In males can occur at any age

Q4.53 Following a colon resection a 70-year-old lady of 60 kg with Parkinson's disease became very distressed and unable to get pain relief with morphine infusion pump, dosage 30 mg in 24 hours:

A. The morphine dose was inadequate
B. The absence of L-dopa therapy may prolong intestinal ileus
C. Nasogastric L-dopa will improve pain relief
D. Gastrointestinal transit may be prolonged in treated Parkinson's disease
E. Monoamine oxidase inhibitors are useful to treat this patient's recurrent depression

Q4.54 The following are characteristic features of irritable bowel syndrome (IBS):

A. Mucus per rectum
B. Diarrhoea
C. Rectal bleeding
D. Weight loss
E. Abdominal pain

Q4.55 The following statements are true of large bowel carcinoma:

A. Rectal bleeding is an early symptom
B. Changes in bowel habit are more frequent in left colonic lesions
C. Males are more commonly affected than females
D. 75% of all cancers are within the reach of a flexible sigmoidoscope
E. Delay in diagnosis is the most significant factor in poor prognosis

Q4.56 Elevated carcino-embryonic antigen (CEA) can be found in the following conditions:

A. Ulcerative colitis without associated colonic cancer
B. Alcoholic hepatitis
C. Lung carcinoma
D. Breast carcinoma
E. Colonic diverticular disease

Q4.57 Folinic acid:

A. Is the acetyl derivative of tetrahydrofolic acid
B. Has a place in the management of advanced colorectal cancer
C. Enhances the anti-tumour efficacy of 5-fluorouracil
D. Leads to the formation of a stable complex with fluorodeoxyuridine monophosphate (F-dUMP) and thymidylate synthetase
E. In combination with 5-fluorouracil is commonly complicated by mucositis

Q4.58 A 35-year-old male with a 15-year history of extensive ulcerative colitis currently in remission maintained on sulpha- salazine 1 g b.d. attends for review:

A. Sulphasalazine should be stopped and changed to one of the newer mesalazine preparations
B. He is at high risk of developing pyoderma gangrenosum
C. He should be advised not to father any children because of the risk of fetal abnormality following the use of sulphasalazine
D. Colonoscopic surveillance is warrented
E. He should have full blood count monitoring

Q4.59 A 22-year-old female gives a two-year history of abdominal distension, frequent loose and urgent stools and crampy hypogastric pains. She has been well investigated and a confident diagnosis of irritable bowel syndrome (IBS) has been made.

A. Approximately one-third of IBS patients have sleep disturbance because of their symptoms
B. Her use of mefenamic acid for dysmenorrhoea, for 7 days each month, could account for her problem
C. It would be appropriate to advise a trial of high fibre diet before recommending specific treatments
D. The long-term use of codeine to control her symptoms could result in opiate addiction
E. The majority of such patients suffer from faecal incontinence, which may not be reported

4. Answers

A4.1
A. True
B. False
C. True
D. False
E. True

Yersinia enterocolitica infection causes an acute enteritic syndrome lasting one to two weeks. Persistent inflammatory changes in the distal ileum have been reported, but strictures and fistula do not occur. Acute appendiceal inflammation and mesenteric lymphadenitis may occur. The bacteria has beta-lactamase activity and is resistant to penicillin, but sensitive to ciprofloxacin, tetracycline and trimethoprim-sulphamethoxazole. Increased host iron stores have been associated with a greater risk of infection with *Yersinia*.

A4.2
A. True
B. True
C. False
D. True
E. True

Antibiotic diarrhoea is common, but after prolonged treatment there is a substantial risk of pseudo-membranous colitis caused by *Clostridium difficile* infection. This can be very serious. If this infection can be proved then specific treatment should be given, preferably by mouth, but the response is not always good.

A4.3
A. True
B. True
C. False
D. True
E. False

Ischaemic colitis can present as acute severe ischaemia or as non-gangrenous colitis with resolution. More than 50% of cases are due to atherosclerotic disease of the mesenteric vessels, often in elderly patients with pre-existing cardiac disease. However, young persons may also be affected, especially those using the oral contraceptive pill and in athletes running long distances. Some histological features are more typical of ischaemic colitis than inflammatory bowel disease, such as a lack of chronic inflammatory cells and the presence of haemosiderin-laden macrophages in the lamina propria. Radiological features of ischaemic colitis include thumb printing, saw-toothing, tubular narrowing and thickening of mucosal folds. Dilatation of the colon may involve the area of ischaemia, or occur proximal to the area of ischaemia or involve the entire colon.

A4.4

A. False
B. True
C. False
D. False
E. False

The majority of cases may be successfully managed with medical treatment. Colectomy is reserved for severe refractory symptoms and persistent dysplasia on biopsy, and sometimes for actual carcinoma of the colon.

A4.5

A. True
B. True
C. False
D. False
E. True

Collagenous colitis presents as chronic watery diarrhoea in women in their sixth and seventh decades. Auto-immune diseases such as rheumatoid arthritis, systemic sclerosis, CREST syndrome and Sjögren's syndrome may be associated. A thickened sub-epithelial collagen plate is diagnostic, and microscopic inflammation with increased intra-epithelial and lamina propria lymphocytes is present. Faecal stream diversion may improve symptoms and reduce the thickness of the sub-epithelial collagen layer. Colonic changes may be patchy and confined to the proximal colon.

A4.6

A. True
B. True
C. True
D. True
E. False

Non-neoplastic polyps are either metaplastic polyps which are typically sessile, round, smooth lesions and less than one cm in size, or pseudo-polyps which are associated with colonic inflammation. Malignant change is found in roughly 10% of adenomas between 1 cm and 2 cm in size. Induration of the lesion or its base would suggest malignancy. Colorectal polyps are often multiple and carcinomas often co-exist with benign tumours. Since there is a risk of malignancy total excision biopsy is performed if possible. Usually a small pedunculated polyp can be removed endoscopically with a diathermy snare. Lower rectal polyps can be excised under general anaesthetic via the anal canal. Only if residual malignancy is proven after biopsy excision should anterior resection be carried out for such a polyp in the upper rectum.

A4.7
A. False
B. True
C. True
D. True
E. True

Acute appendicitis is misdiagnosed in a large minority of cases. Laparoscopy, ultrasonography and even CT/MRI scanning have been proposed to reduce the rate of unnecessary surgery. Crohn's disease can masquerade as acute appendicitis. Removal of the appendix may alter immune function, and is definitely less common as a past medical history in patients with ulcerative colitis. The rise in appendicectomy followed the development of safe abdominal surgery – cases of appendicitis may well have been missed before.

A4.8
A. False
B. True
C. True
D. True
E. False

The conventional regime involves stopping oral feeding, intravenous fluids, high dose steroids, aminosalicylates, antibiotics and transfusion as required. Oral immunosuppressants are not effective.

It is sometimes useful to try intravenous cyclosporin 4 mg/kg/day for a week if patients do not respond in three days.

The need for stopping oral feeding has been questioned and it may be that this can be permitted. Lactose intolerance may be a factor in a minority of patients, however.

Heparin has specific anti-inflammatory actions as well as protecting from thromboembolism. If surgery is needed then a panproctocolectomy is the standard procedure.

A4.9
A. False
B. True
C. True
D. False
E. True

Appropriate surgery is the basic treatment, but results can be improved by adjuvant radiotherapy and chemotherapy. The usual treatment is a combination of 5-fluorouracil plus folinic acid, but ralitrexed is a reserve where these cannot be used.

A4.10
A. True
B. False
C. False
D. True
E. False

Ulcerative colitis and Crohn's disease are genetically associated. There is familial aggregation, so that relatives of an index case are more likely to suffer from some sort of inflammatory bowel disease too than the rest of the population. This tendency is most strong for Crohn's disease in identical twins. The overall prevalence of inflammatory bowel disease in Western societies is about 1 in 500 now. It has been suggested that clinical presentations are increased by the wide use of NSAID therapy causing colitis.

A4.11
A. True
B. True
C. False
D. True
E. True

A4.12
A. True
B. True
C. True
D. False
E. True

Specific associations of chemotherapy for cancer include neutropenic enterocolitis and *Clostridium difficile* pseudomembranous colitis. Neutropenic patients will be more prone to infections of various types, but giardiasis is generally a small bowel disease. Ulcerative colitis could be the problem, but would be a co-incidental illness.

A4.13
A. True
B. False
C. True
D. False
E. True

The likely diagnosis is ulcerative colitis or diverticular disease, but carcinoma needs to be excluded by barium enema or colonoscopy. Flexible sigmoidoscopy is a simple out-patient investigation which will be able to identify ulcerative colitis and most large bowel carcinomas. Biopsy histology is crucial in management. In ulcerative colitis there is characteristic superficial inflammation, goblet cell depletion and crypt abscesses. Surgery is only needed in a minority of ulcerative colitis cases.

A4.14
A. True
B. True
C. True
D. False
E. False

X-ray treatment and fluorouracil combinations improve outcome. If colostomy or ileostomy are performed counselling should precede surgery.

A4.15
A. False
B. False
C. True
D. False
E. True

Butyrate is the main energy source in the colon and promotes cell proliferation. Glutamine is an energy source in the small bowel. Short chain fatty acids such as butyrate are avidly absorbed by the colonic epithelium, and diversion of the faecal stream may lead to colitis due to lack of butyrate. Bile acids cannot be absorbed by colonic epithelium and promote water and electrolyte secretion leading to watery diarrhoea.

A4.16
A. False
B. True
C. True
D. False
E. False

Carcinoma of the rectum and colon is less common than lung carcinoma. There is a definite familial tendency, which can sometimes be identified by searching for oncogenes, but is generally detectable by history taking. Though there is increased risk of malignancy in ulcerative colitis and especially in familial polyposis of the colon, these comprise only a tiny fraction of large bowel carcinoma cases. The condition is usually at an advanced stage when diagnosis is made so that surgery is not usually curative.

A4.17
A. True
B. True
C. False
D. True
E. False
Aminosalicylates such as mesalazine are effective in all forms of ulcerative colitis and colonic Crohn's disease. Though topical steroids are very useful, systemic treatment with prednisolone or azathioprine can also be needed. Sometimes refractory disease requires surgery, and normally a panprocto-colectomy is performed. Ileal pouch operations may be useful, but the patient must be prepared for an ileostomy.

A4.18
A. True
B. True
C. False
D. False
E. True
Radiation damage to the gut may be early, when the effect is mainly on the intestinal epithelium, or late, when the vascular endothelium is progressively affected leading to occlusion of the blood vessels. Rectovaginal fistula is a well known complication of radiotherapy and characterised by faecal leakage and perineal discomfort. Intestinal stricture formation is a late sequel of radiation induced vascular damage – concurrent chemotherapy, previous pelvic surgery and diabetes, hypertension and atherosclerosis may favour the development of radiation bowel disease. During radiotherapy, meganucleosis, eosinophilic abscess and oedema of the lamina propria may occur. Radiation bowel disease may continue to progress even after surgical defunctioning.

A4.19
A. True
B. True
C. True
D. True
E. True

A4.20
A. True
B. False
C. True
D. True
E. True

The most probable diagnosis is 'pouchitis'. This is likely to affect about a third of patients within five years after RPC for ulcerative colitis. The cause is unknown but suggested factors are bacterial overgrowth, stasis and ischaemia. *Clostridium difficile* is not the cause of pouchitis itself but it and other acute gut pathogens should be sought in this patient by stool culture. In some patients pouchitis may represent undiagnosed Crohn's disease. A rapid response to metronidazole is almost diagnostic of pouchitis. It is effective in 80–90% of patients.

A4.21
A. False
B. True
C. True
D. True
E. True

A4.22
A. False
B. True
C. True
D. True
E. True

This rare condition typically causes watery profuse secretory diarrhoea in middle-aged women. Colonoscopy is usually normal but biopsy demonstrates an abnormal sub-epithelial band of type III collagen. Amino-salicylates, steroids and surgery have all been used in treatment.

A4.23
A. False
B. True
C. True
D. True
E. True

A4.24
A. False
B. True
C. True
D. False
E. True

A4.25
A. False
B. False
C. True
D. False
E. False

The pain in IBS can occur anywhere in the abdomen and is usually relieved by defecation. Weight loss would suggest a more sinister pathology and an increased mucosal vascular pattern is an early sign of inflammatory change. With typical symptoms and nothing else to suggest organic disease radiology is not required.

A4.26
A. True
B. False
C. True
D. False
E. False

A4.27
A. False
B. False
C. True
D. False
E. False

Defective pelvic floor function leads to obstructing prolapse of rectal mucosa during defecation with ischaemia, ulceration and bleeding. Although self-digitation may be used to relieve the obstruction and allow stool passage, it is now discredited as a cause of ulceration. The combination of changes of prolapse with ischaemia and superficial ulceration are felt to be characteristic on histology.

A4.28
A. False
B. False
C. False
D. False
E. False

A4.29
A. False
B. False
C. True
D. False
E. True

Familial adenomatous polyposis usually does not cause symptoms until teenage or early adult life. However, with more widespread screening of high-risk individuals the disease may be diagnosed before the onset of symptoms. In FAP polyps have been demonstrated in the small bowel and stomach. Hereditary non-polyposis colon cancer (HNPCC) (Lynch syndrome) is more common than FAP. HNPCC is responsible for 5% of all colon cancers whereas FAP is responsible for 0.5% of all colon cancers. The risk of colon cancer in FAP increases with age. Colectomy is usually performed at 15 to 20 years of age.

A4.30
A. True
B. True
C. False
D. False
E. False

A4.31
A. False
B. False
C. True
D. False
E. True

Occasionally hair loss is a drug-related phenomenon. It can accompany mental stress. Recovery from illness may be a cause of hair loss but is followed by more vigorous regrowth.

A4.32

A. True
B. True
C. False
D. True
E. False

Crohn's disease and ulcerative colitis need consideration. The commonest associated liver disease is primary sclerosing cholangitis in ulcerative colitis, but chronic autoimmune hepatitis, primary biliary cirrhosis, amyloid and liver abscesses are all linked in addition. Metastatic carcinoma of the rectum is a contender for the diagnosis despite relatively young age because it is such a common condition. Biopsy of the tumour and/or the liver should yield a diagnosis. Underlying inflammatory bowel disease may explain premature malignant disease, which is a recognised complication.

A4.33

A. True
B. True
C. True
D. True
E. False

A4.34

A. True
B. True
C. False
D. False
E. True

First-degree relatives of patients with colon carcinoma have a two-to-three-fold increased risk of colon cancer, and the relative risk is increased to three-to-six-fold above the population risk if two or more relatives are affected or if a first degree relative is diagnosed at an age of 50 years or less. Metaplastic polyps are not associated with neoplastic change. Adenomata need to be screened for one year after a 'clean colon' has been achieved. The indications for surveillance screening in Crohn's colitis are not as clearly agreed as in UC, but long-standing total Crohn's colitis carries a significant risk of neoplastic transformation. One-off *flexible sigmoidoscopy* has been proposed as a cost-effective measure to screen for colorectal carcinoma in the general population, but it is not yet officially recommended in the UK.

A4.35
A. True
B. False
C. True
D. True
E. True

A4.36
A. True
B. False
C. True
D. True
E. True

Asymptomatic *Clostridium difficile* is present in many healthy people and carriage is increased in ulcerative colitis. It increases in frequency after a variety of antibiotics, and in some is associated with diarrhoea. In a small minority of cases the patient becomes febrile and toxic with bloody diarrhoea and this is associated with pseudomembranous colitis. Treatment with metronidazole or vancomycin is useful but does not always work. The elderly are a particular risk population.

A4.37
A. False
B. False
C. False
D. False
E. False

A4.38
A. False
B. True
C. True
D. False
E. True

In 1987 there were over 28 000 new cases of colorectal cancer in the United Kingdom and in 1991 there were some 19 000 deaths. Colorectal cancer is the second most common cause of cancer death after lung cancer. Overall rates of 'curative' resection vary widely. Over 20% of patients present with distant metastases. At present most authorities would recommend adjuvant chemotherapy (usually with 5-fluorouracil (5-FU) and folinic acid) in Dukes C stage tumours, but there remains controversy over its use in Dukes B cases.

A4.39
A. False
B. False
C. True
D. False
E. True

Recto-sigmoid polyps are common, and there is a definite potential for malignancy in those larger than 10 mm, so removal is advisable. They may be associated with polyps or carcinoma elsewhere in the large bowel so complete evaluation is required to plan management properly.

A4.40
A. True
B. True
C. True
D. True
E. False

A4.41
A. True
B. False
C. True
D. True
E. True

Ulcerative colitis and two-thirds of large bowel carcinomas will be detected by flexible sigmoidoscopy to the splenic flexure/transverse colon. Barium enema or colonoscopy are needed as well for completeness, but vigorous bowel preparation is important to avoid errors. Mucosal lesions such as angiodysplasia are only apparent to direct vision and will not show on barium radiology. Where other tests have failed or are impossible, computed tomography scanning is helpful.

A4.42
A. False
B. False
C. True
D. True
E. True

Pneumatosis coli is an uncommon condition which is usually idiopathic. It can involve large and small bowel, but generally spares the rectum. It can be asymptomatic or present with diarrhoea and bleeding.

A4.43

A. True
B. False
C. True
D. False
E. False

5-ASA compounds are effective in maintaining remission and treating relapses in mild to moderate disease. *Irreversible* nephritis is a side-effect of mesalazine. Azathioprine is effective in maintaining a remission in Crohn's disease but can take several months to exert its effect.

A4.44

A. False
B. False
C. False
D. False
E. True

This lady, who had had her ileo-caecal valve removed in the course of this resection, had bile salt diarrhoea, and was rendered symptom-free after 40 years' diarrhoea by taking cholestyramine.

A4.45

A. False
B. True
C. False
D. False
E. False

This man has a localised colitis with mild symptoms, and it is very likely that he will respond to rectal steroids. Intravenous steroids would mean admitting him to hospital, and it is unlikely that this is necessary. Cyclosporin may rarely be helpful in some patients with severe resistant proctitis but causes unpleasant side-effects and is not indicated here.

A4.46

A. False
B. True
C. False
D. False
E. False

Abdominal bloating is a common complaint in functional bowel disorders. Blood mixed with the stool should not be ascribed to haemorrhoidal bleeding and warrants further investigation. Anti-depressants such as the tricyclics are used in some cases of functional bowel disorder, not specifically for their anti-depressant effect but also because of their effects on motility and pain perception. However, they are not normally used first line.

A4.47
A. False
B. False
C. True
D. False
E. True
Steroid enemas do result in steroid absorption and can cause adrenal suppression. Liquid enemas reach the splenic flexure, foam enemas to approximately the sigmoid colon and suppositories remain in the rectum. A recent meta-analysis suggests mesalazine enemas are more effective than steroid enemas in inducing remission of distal ulcerative colitis. Although there is an increased risk of bowel malignancy in patients with extensive colitis of more than 10 years duration, there is no scientific evidence that endoscopic surveillance reduces mortality. Acute renal failure is a reported complication of mesalazine.

A4.48
A. False
B. False
C. True
D. False
E. True
The approximate lifetime risk of colonic cancer in the general population is 1 in 50 and in a patient with a first-degree relative developing cancer of the colon and age > 45 is 1 in 17.

A4.49
A. False
B. True
C. True
D. False
E. True
Radiotherapy for pelvic lesions damages the ileum most commonly, as it is less free to move during a radiotherapy course. Histology shows endarteritis and fibrosis of the bowel wall. The site of the fistula, any discontinuity of the bowel, abscess formation or distal obstruction must be determined, and this is best done by a sinogram. Good nutrition, skin care and eventual resection and anastomosis clear of radiotherapy damaged bowel is essential for a successful outcome.

A4.50
A. False
B. True
C. True
D. False
E. True

Although carcinoma of the colon may recur 4 years after surgery, the patient being symptomless until recent diarrhoea makes non-malignant reason likely. Diarrhoea and weight loss without vomiting with air in the colon means the anastomosis is likely to be patent. The cause of the diarrhoea is probably small bowel obstruction with bacterial overgrowth, all of which may be cured by surgical adesiolysis.

A4.51
A. False
B. True
C. False
D. False
E. True

This lady with known diverticular disease almost certainly has a pericolic abscess, with small bowel adherence to the abscess wall causing small bowel obstruction. Barium enema in the acute stage is dangerous and would not show the small bowel obstruction. Intravenous fluids, antibiotics and nasogastric section may resolve the situation. Continued small bowel obstruction, increased tenderness and toxicity are indications for surgical management. This may just require laparotomy and small bowel adhesiolysis, but if the pericolic abscess has a visible communication with the large bowel lumen then resection of the large bowel with Hartmann procedure and colostomy is needed. In very experienced surgical hands acute large bowel resection and anastomosis may be attempted.

A4.52
A. False
B. False
C. True
D. True
E. True

The combination of uterovaginal and rectal prolapse is relatively infrequent. Most patients with full thickness rectal prolapse have a history of faecal incontinence. In gross rectal prolapse the diagnosis is usually clear, but lesser degrees of complete prolapse may be difficult to distinguish on inspection alone from mucosal prolapse or prolapse of haemorrhoids. Profound laxity of the sphincters would suggest a complete rectal prolapse.

A4.53
A. **False**
B. **False**
C. **True**
D. **True**
E. **False**

A nasogastric tube can be used Parkinson's disease over abdominal surgery to infuse liquid or powdered anti-Parkinsonian treatment into the gastrointestinal tract. The prevention of increasing muscular tone will aid pain relief from an abdominal wound. Anticholinergics cause slowed motility and in an old patient they may still be given but are now rarely used. Monoamine oxidase inhibitors are contra-indicated with L-dopa/carbidopa.

A4.54
A. **True**
B. **True**
C. **False**
D. **False**
E. **True**

The six symptoms which best characterise IBS are abdominal pain relieved by defecation, looser and more frequent stools at the onset of abdominal pain, distention, mucus and a feeling of incomplete rectal evacuation (the Manning criteria).

A4.55
A. **False**
B. **True**
C. **False**
D. **True**
E. **True**

In right-sided lesions patients may present with iron deficiency anaemia only. Colonic cancer affects men and women equally. As tumours start showing evidence of spread to regional lymph nodes even when the local involvement is only sub-mucosal surgery is very often not curative.

A4.56
A. **True**
B. **True**
C. **True**
D. **True**
E. **False**

CEA is a non-specific marker which is raised in a wide variety of benign diseases and also in malignancies, in particular, the entodermally derived neoplasms of the gastrointestinal tract and lungs. It is also useful to monitor colonic cancer following surgical resection if present prior to surgery.

A4.57

A. False
B. True
C. True
D. True
E. True

Folinic acid is the formyl derivative of tetrahydrofolic acid. It has been used in combination with 5-fluorouracil (5-FU), in the therapy of advanced colorectal cancer and also in adjuvant therapy in some resected cases. Folinic acid is thought to modulate the biochemical activity of 5-FU. The plasma half-life of 5-FU after intravenous bolus administration is about 10 minutes. Addition of folinic acid increases the formation and stability of the fluorodeoxyuridylate–thymidylate synthetase complex which increases the active half-life to about 18 hours. This increases the cytotoxic activity of the 5-FU. Mucositis is a common toxic effect seen in colorectal cancer patients receiving 5-FU and folinic acid. It may be decreased by sucking ice chips, starting five minutes before each dose of 5-FU. Other important toxic effects of this drug combination are diarrhoea and leucopenia.

A4.58

A. False
B. False
C. False
D. True
E. True

A4.59

A. False
B. True
C. False
D. True
E. False

Sleep disturbance during sleep is unusual in IBS and should prompt suspicions of organic disease. 'Pseudo-IBS', secondary to NSAIDs (and other drugs such as proton pump inhibitors, iron supplements, opiate painkillers, agents with anti-cholinergic effects, antibiotics and lipid lowering agents) is common. The only symptom likely to improve with increased fibre intake is constipation: bloating and urgent diarrhoea will be aggravated. Codeine is inappropriate for long-term use in this situation: loperamide is safe and effective. Incontinence is the (often unvoiced) reason for seeking advice in about 20% of patients like this.

5. Liver and Spleen

Q5.1 **An 82-year-old man was admitted with jaundice, abdominal pain and hepatomegaly with a central boss. Serum is positive for hepatitis C by ELISA and RIBA. He was formerly a heavy drinker but denied drug abuse.**

A. He could have been infected by tattooing
B. Blood transfusion could have been the route of transmission
C. Sexual transmission needs to be considered
D. HCV may have been present for many years
E. There could be both cirrhosis and hepatoma

Q5.2 **The quadrate lobe of the liver:**

A. Is otherwise known as segment IV
B. Is part of the right hemi-liver
C. Can be excised to allow adequate resection of a hilar cholangio-carcinoma
D. Derives its blood supply mainly from the portal vein
E. Lies to the right of the ligamentum teres

Q5.3 **In a jaundiced patient, an extrahepatic cause is suggested by:**

A. Scratch marks
B. Palmar erythema
C. Palpable gallbladder
D. Facial telangiectasia
E. Dilated common bile duct on ultrasonography

Q5.4 **In cirrhotic ascites:**

A. The total body sodium is low
B. A low sodium diet is indicated
C. Urinary sodium excretion is reduced
D. Intravenous saline is indicated if plasma sodium falls below 115 mmol/l
E. Diuretic treatment should aim for a fluid loss of two litres daily

Q5.5   Medically important increasing alcohol consumption is seen in:

A. UK
B. USA
C. France
D. Women
E. Saudi Arabia

Q5.6   Important signs of hepatocellular failure are:

A. Campbell de Morgan spots
B. Spider naevi
C. Palmar erythema
D. White nails
E. Jaundice

Q5.7   Chronic hepatitis is sometimes a side-effect of:

A. Captopril
B. Methyldopa
C. Isoniazid
D. Ethambutol
E. Dantrolene

Q5.8   In hepatitis C infection:

A. Liver function tests are a useful guide to histological stage
B. Infection acquired through intravenous drug abuse is associated with a
   worse prognosis than after blood transfusion
C. The initial infection is usually asymptomatic
D. Most individuals clear the virus
E. Interferon treatment produces permanent clearance of the virus in only
   25% of those treated

**Q5.9   Common causes of cirrhosis are alcohol, viruses and auto-
         immune disease. Other reasons are:**

A. Lead poisoning
B. Herbal teas with *Senecio* and *Crotalaria*
C. Chronic biliary obstruction
D. Glycogen storage disease
E. Gallbladder stones

Q5.10 Liver abscess:

A. Generally is blood-borne via the hepatic artery
B. Is often related to cholangitis
C. Is associated with Crohn's disease
D. Can be cured by metronidazole, if amoebic
E. Is invariably fatal

Q5.11 A 48-year-old female with ulcerative colitis develops severe episodic painful jaundice. Abdominal ultrasonography is normal. Tests likely to give a diagnosis are:

A. Oral cholecystogram
B. Endoscopic retrograde cholangiopancreatography (ERCP)
C. Mitochondrial antibody
D. Perinuclear anti-neutrophil cytoplasmic antibody (pANCA)
E. Liver biopsy

Q5.12 Primary liver cell carcinoma is caused by:

A. Hepatitis A
B. Hepatitis B
C. Hepatitis C
D. Alcohol
E. Aflatoxin

Q5.13 Portal hypertension may be a feature in:

A. Constrictive pericarditis
B. Inferior vena cava obstruction
C. Alcoholic central hyaline necrosis
D. Vitamin A poisoning
E. Sarcoidosis

Q5.14 A 75-year-old woman was admitted to hospital with a treated lower respiratory tract infection. Routine blood tests showed elevated bilirubin, markedly elevated glutamyl transferase, alkaline phosphatase and ALT levels. Albumin was normal as was a haemogram.

A. This could all be a non-specific associate of a chest infection and resolve spontaneously
B. Common bile duct gallstone disease could co-exist
C. There may be separate viral liver disease
D. Prior amoxycillin therapy would explain the problem
E. She may have autoimmune hepatitis

Q5.15 A 70-year-old man on a programme of venesection for haemochromatosis develops jaundice with itching, dark urine and pale diarrhoea.

A. This could be cirrhosis
B. Hepatoma may have developed
C. Gallstones in the common bile duct could explain the problem
D. Pancreatic carcinoma may have occurred
E. Treatment with low fat diet and cholestyramine will give symptomatic relief

Q5.16 A 20-year-old male is the partner of a woman with acute hepatitis B. He is known to be HBsAg negative and susceptible to the disease:

A. He should be given human immunoglobulins
B. He should receive rapid immunisation with 3 injections at monthly intervals
C. He should use condoms until proved immune
D. Their children aged 2 and 5 are at risk
E. She will have a 90% chance of developing lifelong hepatitis B virus immunity, but may also be co-infected with HIV

Q5.17 A 58-year-old woman attended clinic with hepatomegaly and marked ascites. No clear alcohol history was obtainable and she had no relevant family history. Serum ferritin was markedly raised and she was found to have diabetes mellitus:

A. Laparoscopic liver biopsy is needed
B. Family screening may be required
C. This could be cirrhosis with hepatoma
D. Wilson's disease could be the problem
E. Haemochromatosis is possible

Q5.18 Hepatitis C infection is:

A. Usually a chronic problem
B. Can lead to cirrhosis and hepatoma
C. Is transmitted by the faecal–oral route
D. Is commoner in haemophiliacs
E. Is proved by positive ELISA testing

Q5.19 Liver transplantation:

A Requires careful HLA tissue typing to be successful

B. Is indicated in alcoholic liver disease

C. Has an appreciable early mortality but thereafter life expectancy can be normal

D. Achieves better results in primary biliary cirrhosis than primary sclerosing cholangitis

E. Requires prolonged immune suppression therapy

Q5.20 In chronic autoimmune hepatitis:

A. A characteristic abnormality is raised alkaline phosphatase and gamma-glutamyl transferase level

B. Serum mitochondrial antibodies are present

C. Serum immunoglobulin G is elevated

D. Treatment is based on steroids and immunosuppressant therapy

E. Life expectancy is improved by therapy

Q5.21 A 38-year-old man is admitted with confusion, agitation and a new internal squint. His condition worsens and he develops nystagmus. He reports an alcohol intake of 42 units weekly.

A. Intravenous vitamins B and C are useful

B. The alcohol history may be misleading

C. This is Korsakoff psychosis

D. He may continue moderate alcohol intake

E. The problem may be permanent

Q5.22 Adverse prognostic findings on liver biopsy in alcoholism are:

A. Iron deposition

B. Large mitochondria

C. Hepatitis

D. Peri-venular sclerosis

E. Steatosis

Q5.23 Drugs useful in the management of alcoholic liver disease include:

A. Acarbose

B. Acamprosate

C. Acetaldehyde

D. Abciximab

E. Antabuse

Q5.24 Elevation of alkaline phosphatase and glutamyl transferase are characteristic of:

A. Liver metastases
B. Biliary obstruction
C. Acute viral hepatitis
D. Anticonvulsant therapy
E. Gilbert's syndrome

Q5.25 The following antibodies can be found in chronic autoimmune hepatitis (CAIH):

A. Antinuclear antibody (ANA)
B. Anti-smooth muscle antibody (SMA)
C. Anti-mitochondrial antibody (AMA)
D. Liver kidney microsomal antibody (LKM)
E. Rheumatoid factor (RF)

Q5.26 A 25-year-old mother of two children develops acute hepatitis B two months after a termination of pregnancy. She denied intravenous drug abuse and had never been transfused:

A. This illness is likely to be self-limiting
B. If her partner is hepatitis B surface antigen positive he is likely to be the source of infection
C. If her partner is hepatitis B surface antigen negative he should be immunised rapidly
D. Barrier contraception will reduce the risk of transmission
E. The patient should be tested for HIV

Q5.27 A 55-year-old woman from County Durham developed jaundice, ascites, lethargy, pruritus, pale stools and dark urine. After a partial recovery liver biopsy showed cirrhosis. She had had two blood transfusions, 2 and 34 years ago. ELISA anti-HCV test was negative. There was no history of alcohol abuse:

A. This is likely to be autoimmune liver disease
B. A positive HAV IgG test shows that this is hepatitis A
C. In time the liver will return to normal
D. Liver transplantation may be required
E. Interferon-α therapy is useful

Q5.28 A conscious and violent 36-year-old man is brought to hospital in police custody with a history that he has taken 150 tablets of co-proxamol two days before and drinks 10–12 pints of beer daily. 'Liver function' tests show a raised glutamyl transferase level of 85 IU/l, but are otherwise normal. Drug screen is negative for paracetamol and other agents though there is alcohol present:

A. Patient should receive immediate acetylcysteine infusion
B. Alcohol withdrawal symptoms may be a problem
C. Respiratory depression could occur
D. If there are no fresh medical problems after observation for a few hours he should return to custody
E. Liver damage could still occur

Q5.29 Fever, lymphadenopathy, abnormal 'liver function' tests and splenomegaly in a young man raise the possibility of:

A. Infectious mononucleosis
B. Toxoplasmosis
C. Malaria
D. AIDS
E. Lymphoma

Q5.30 A 34-year-old man is admitted with a 3-week history of increasing painless jaundice. He had been drinking heavily for the past three years – latterly one bottle of vodka daily. He had just returned from six weeks in Greece. He had 5 cm hepatomegaly and slight fever, no other abnormal findings. Bilirubin 680 μmol/l, alk phos 3692 U/l, γGT 4709 U/l, AST 210 U/l, ALT 98 U/l, albumin 22 g/l, globulin 28 g/l. Prothrombin time was 13 s. Ultrasonography showed hepatomegaly and a uniform fine bright echo pattern, biliary tree normal. Testing for hepatitis A associated IgM, BHsAg and hepatitis C antibody is negative:

A. He does not have acute alcoholic hepatitis
B. He does not have acute hepatitis B
C. He cannot have acute hepatitis C
D. He is at high risk of developing delirium tremens
E. Steps should be taken to prevent the development of encephalopathy

Q5.31 A 58-year-old teacher was admitted with increasing jaundice and a weight loss of 6 kg over the last 3 months, on two occasions he had noticed dark motions which cleared within two days following which his stools looked abnormally pale. He had no episodes of chills or rigors. His past medical history included Billroth I gastrectomy for peptic ulcer 26 years ago. He smoked 15 cigarettes a day and drank about 20 units of spirits a week. His haemoglobin was 8.6 g/dl, bilirubin 196 μmol/l, alkaline phosphatase 842 units/l, ALT 112 units/l, albumin 39 g/l. US scan abdomen showed dilated biliary tree. Differential diagnosis would include:

A. Alcoholic liver disease
B. Gastric cancer
C. Pancreatic cancer
D. Choledocholithiasis
E. Carcinoma of the ampulla of Vater

Q5.32 Which of the following are true in liver disease:

A. Bleeding is always corrected by vitamin K
B. Bleeding may follow biliary obstruction
C. Thrombocytopenia would be an unexpected finding
D. The prothrombin time is an adequate test
E. Vitamin K dependent factors and liver factors are synonymous

Q5.33 In primary biliary cirrhosis:

A. The titre of antimitochondrial antibody correlates with the stage of the disease
B. The bile ducts are destroyed by B-lymphocytes
C. The mitochondrial auto-antigen includes pyruvate dehydrogenase complex
D. Colchicine produces significant histological improvement
E. Renal tubular defects may exist

Q5.34 The fact that the caudate lobe of the liver has an independent venous drainage is significant in which of the following conditions:

A. Acute liver failure
B. Primary biliary cirrhosis
C. Budd–Chiari syndrome
D. Haemochromatosis
E. Wilson's disease

Q5.35 In Wilson's disease:

A. The cause is a deficiency of caeruloplasmin
B. Neurological presentation is common in the first decade
C. Presentation may be with an acute haemolytic anaemia
D. Raised 24 hour urinary copper excretion is pathognomonic
E. The treatment of choice is triethyl tetramine dihydrochloride (trientine)

Q5.36 Hepatitis C:

A. Is decreasing in prevalence in the UK
B. Has a better prognosis if linked with a high viral load
C. Sub-typing may be useful for prognosis
D. Liver histology may be abnormal even if LFTs are normal
E. Cirrhosis is linked with poor response to therapy

Q5.37 With regard to alcoholic liver function:

A. There is a good relationship between ultrasound appearance and bio-chemistry
B. The extent of histological damage is predictable from the level of alcohol consumption
C. Alcoholic patients are often hypertensive on benzodiazepine sedation
D. Fatty infiltration is usually only seen in end-stage liver disease
E. The transaminase levels are usually the best test of liver synthetic function

Q5.38 Ursodeoxycholic acid is officially licensed for treatment of:

A. Steatorrhoea
B. Gallstone dissolution
C. Chronic pancreatitis
D. Primary biliary cirrhosis
E. Hepatitis B

Q5.39 In hepatocellular carcinoma:

A. Increasing concentrations of circulating α-fetoprotein are a manifestation of carcino-foetal reversion
B. Prognosis is dependent principally on tumour size with lesions less than 2 cm having a reasonable chance of cure
C. Circulating α-fetoprotein is detectable in normal adult serum
D. Circulating α-fetoprotein may be elevated in the regenerative phase of viral hepatitis
E. Circulating α-fetoprotein may be elevated in 15% of cirrhotic patients

Q5.40 In the pharmacotherapy of portal hypertension:

A. Nitrates increase the cardiac index but reduce portal pressure
B. β-Blockers increase the cardiac index but reduce portal pressure
C. Selective β-blockers have the same efficacy at portal pressure reduction as less selective ones
D. The addition of nitrates to beta-blockers can reduce the unwanted effects of beta-blockade
E. β-Blockers reduce the incidence and mortality of acute variceal bleeding

Q5.41 A patient with portosystemic encephalopathy is confused and noisy. In an attempt to control the symptoms should the patient be given:

A. Morphine
B. Diazepam
C. Paraldehyde
D. Low protein diet
E. Neomycin

Q5.42 *N*-acetylcysteine:

A. Reduces the production of the *N*-acetyl-*p*-benzoquinoneimine metabolite of paracetamol
B. 70% is renally excreted in man
C. When given to the at-risk population defined as those with plasma paracetamol concentrations above a semi-logarithmic plot of 200 mg/l at 4 hours and 30 mg/l at 15 hours prevents significant liver disease
D. Blocks electrophiles and scavenges reactive oxygen species
E. Is of greater value in late than early paracetamol poisoning

Q5.43 A 45-year-old lady developed fulminant hepatic failure which may have been secondary to diclofenac. Hepatic damage from non-steroidal drugs:

A. Is most common in women and in those over 50 years of age
B. Is more common in those with underlying autoimmune disease
C. Can have serological and histological features of autoimmune chronic active hepatitis
D. Occurs on rechallenge with the drug
E. Most often occurs due to hypersensitivity

Q5.44 In paracetamol poisoning the degree of liver injury is dependent upon:

A. The total quantity and rate of paracetamol absorbed
B. The metabolic activity of cytochrome P450 mixed function oxidase
C. Rate of elimination and disposition of the toxic and non-toxic paracetamol metabolites
D. The amount and rate of regeneration of hepatic glutathione
E. The weight of the patient

Q5.45 Liver orcein stains demonstrate:

A. Hepatitis A virus in hepatocytes
B. Hepatitis B virus in hepatocytes
C. Hepatitis C virus in hepatocytes
D. Copper binding protein
E. Cellular iron

Q5.46 In autoimmune chronic active hepatitis (CAIH) type I with nuclear and smooth muscle antibodies:

A. Azathioprine is the treatment of choice for severe relapses
B. Azathioprine can be used alone to maintain remission
C. Withdrawal of treatment should be considered after six months of remission
D. Patients who have had withdrawal of treatment after five years of remission need to be followed up every three months indefinitely
E. There is an association with hepatitis C virus

Q5.47 In untreated patients with cirrhosis due to hereditary haemochromatosis:

A. Adequate iron removal normalises the risk of subsequent hepatocellular carcinoma development
B. Adequate iron removal normalises the associated hormonal abnormalities
C. Cardiac failure may be the presenting complaint
D. The treatment of choice is intravenous desferrioxamine
E. A previous history of excessive beer drinking is often elicited

Q5.48 Jaundice associated with a high level of unconjugated bilirubin in the serum may occur in:

A. Haemolytic anaemia
B. Some types of ineffective erythropoiesis
C. Excessive eating
D. Gilbert's syndrome
E. Rotor syndrome

Q5.49 A 20-year-old woman presents with abdominal pain and nausea 30 hours after ingestion of 50 g of paracetamol. She is slightly drowsy. Serum bilirubin is 32 mol/l (upper limit of normal 18 mol/l) and AST > 4000 IU/l. Prothrombin time is 35 s (control 12 s) and arterial pH is 7.22:

A. The greatly elevated AST is the most worrisome prognostic feature
B. Advice from a liver unit, with a view to urgent transfer for consideration of liver transplantation, should be urgently sought
C. She has presented too late to benefit from *N*-acetylcysteine
D. Insertion of a central line is inadvisable due to her coagulopathy
E. Lactulose and neomycin would be expected to improve her encephalopathy

Q5.50 In the pathogenesis of hepatocellular carcinoma (HCC):

A. Cirrhosis is the major premalignant lesion
B. Site-specific hepatitis B viral integration activating cellular oncogenes is a common cause of HBV-associated HCC
C. The hepatitis B virus is directly oncogenic
D. Hepatitis C virus has classic flaviviral oncogenic properties
E. Primary biliary cirrhosis is especially implicated by epidemiological studies

Q5.51 Interferon-α treatment is indicated in:

A. AIDS
B. Acute hepatitis B
C. Acute hepatitis A
D. Acute hepatitis D
E. Hepatitis B e antibody carriers

Q5.52 A 55-year-old woman developed painless jaundice over a period of one week. She had a cholecystectomy 5 years previously and had received co-amoxiclav (Augmentin) 5 weeks previously. Liver biochemistry showed bilirubin 350 mol/l, alkaline phosphatase of 600 IU/l (upper limit of normal 170 IU/l), alanine aminotransferase 310 IU/l (10–35 IU/l). Abdominal ultrasonography showed a normal liver texture; the common bile duct diameter was 8 mm and no stones were seen.

A. She should undergo ERCP to exclude extrahepatic biliary obstruction
B. Bilirubin will be mainly unconjugated
C. Her jaundice may be due to co-amoxiclav
D. Allowing for her cholecystectomy, the common bile duct is significantly dilated
E. The clinical presentation is compatible with alcoholic hepatitis

Q5.53 In Wilson's disease (hepatolenticular degeneration):

A. The discovery of the genetic defect responsible has led to the development of tests that can be used for population screening
B. The mutation in the caeruloplasmin gene prevents plasma caeruloplasmin levels reaching normal levels
C. Can be reliably diagnosed by an increased urinary copper excretion
D. Treatment with chelating agents can safely be discontinued after liver biopsy shows no stainable copper
E. Oral zinc is an effective treatment

Q5.54 The use of TIPSS (transvenous intrahepatic portasystem shunt):

A. Can be recommended for bleeding oesophageal varices
B. May be useful for intractable ascites, but not always
C. Is identical in its physiological effects to surgical shunts
D. May cause acute liver failure
E. Leads to improvements in mental function

Q5.55 The following are effective in the treatment of hepatic encephalopathy:

A. Chlordiazepoxide
B. Metronidazole
C. Lactulose
D. Saline infusion
E. Neomycin

Q5.56 Haemochromatosis:

A. Does not occur in women
B. Is autosomal recessive
C. Has its genetic defect located on the same gene as the HLA system
D. Causes decreased intestinal iron absorption
E. Is associated with diabetes mellitus

Q5.57 Survival in alcoholic liver disease:

A. Is not altered in those with fatty liver
B. Is 50% in alcoholic hepatitis
C. Is worse in men than women with cirrhosis
D. Is unrelated to continued alcohol consumption once cirrhosis has developed
E. Is longer than in other forms of cirrhotic liver disease

Q5.58 Histological features of alcoholic liver disease include:

A. Mallory's hyaline
B. Steatosis
C. Granulomas
D. Balloon degeneration
E. Disappearing bile ducts

Q5.59 A 50-year-old lady on HRT presents with jaundice. An abdominal ultrasonogram suggests multiple hepatic second-aries. An ultrasound guided biopsy is negative for malignancy. She stops the HRT and starts to improve clinically and biochemically. Hepatitis markers are all negative. What diagnosis(es) would you entertain:

A. Carcinoma of the breast with liver secondaries
B. Carcinoma of the uterus with liver secondaries
C. Amyloidosis
D. Granulomatous hepatitis
E. Steatosis

Q5.60 A pregnant 25-year-old is found to be hepatitis C virus positive and hepatitis C virus RNA PCR positive:

A. If the LFTs are normal she is non-infectious
B. Acyclovir is the treatment of choice
C. Vertical transmission to the fetus occurs in over 95% of cases
D. Previous blood transfusion is a potential source for her infection
E. She is likely to spontaneously abort

Q5.61 The following immune suppressant drugs are routinely used as primary therapy after liver transplantation:

A. Levamisole
B. Tacrolimus
C. Prednisolone
D. Cyclosporin
E. Azathioprine

Q5.62 The following can be used as markers to monitor chronic alcohol abuse:

A. Glutamyl transferase (GT)
B. Blood alcohol in morning clinics
C. Carbohydrate deficient transferrin (CDT)
D. Serum bilirubin
E. Mean corpuscular volume (MCV)

Q5.63 A patient with cryptogenic hepatic cirrhosis and ascites has suffered from persistent pyrexia for three weeks. The cause may be:

A. Hyperaldosteronism
B. Occult bleeding
C. Hepatoma
D. Liver abscess
E. Peritonitis

Q5.64 A 30-year-old obese woman with two children and no significant past medical history presented with painful jaundice. Ultrasonography showed gallbladder gallstones and ERCP showed normal bile ducts. She had persistent cholestatic jaundice six weeks later with skin itching, pale stools and dark urine. Repeat ultrasonography and ERCP again showed normal bile ducts.

A. This is likely to be chronic *autoimmune* liver disease
B. Alcohol intake needs to be carefully reviewed
C. Percutaneous liver biopsy is indicated
D. Carbon tetrachloride poisoning could explain the problem
E. Carcinoma of the pancreas is in the differential diagnosis

Q5.65 In orthotopic liver transplantation (OLT) for viral hepatitis:

A. Chronic viral hepatitis is the most common indication for this procedure
B. Recurrence of viral hepatitis is a rare event post-operatively
C. In 25% of patients with recurrent viral infection fibrosing cholestatic hepatitis may develop
D. Hepatitis B immunoglobulin (Ig) given prophylactically improves graft survival in those with detectable HBV DNA
E. Viral recurrence after OLT for chronic HCV infection is a more serious event than for HBV

Q5.66 Serum positive for hepatitis A antibody in the IgG class indicates:

A. Recent clinical infection
B. Previous infection
C. Lifelong immunity
D. Continued infectivity
E. Likelihood of hepatoma

Q5.67 Primary sclerosing cholangitis:

A. Involves the gallbladder
B. Predisposes to cholangiocarcinoma
C. Is an autoimmune disease and justifies treatment with steroids and azathioprine
D. May improve following panproctocolectomy
E. Recurs following hepatic transplantation

Q5.68 In patients with liver failure, hepatic encephalopathy:

A. May be precipitated by gastrointestinal haemorrhage
B. May be improved by treatment with lactose
C. May be precipitated by treatment with benzodiazepines
D. Does not occur in drug-induced liver failure
E. May be complicated by cerebral oedema

Q5.69 In a 70-year-old man, newly presenting with gross ascites and jaundice:

A. Liver biopsy is the most useful investigation
B. Laparoscopy may be a valuable management tool
C. If chronic liver disease is diagnosed, it is important to exclude Wilson's disease as a potentially treatable cause
D. Removal of ascites by rapid paracentesis is more hazardous than diuretic therapy
E. If large oesophageal varices are demonstrated, variceal eradication is recommended

Q5.70 In a patient with heart failure:

A. Hepatic encephalopathy may occur in the absence of any other cause of liver disease
B. Dilatation of the portal vein can be demonstrated by ultrasonography
C. Jaundice may occur even in the absence of a raised JVP
D. Weight loss is normally the result of steatorrhoea
E. Dyspnoea correlates well with liver function

Q5.71 In a patient with severe hepatic failure secondary to paracetamol toxicity:

A. Hypoglycaemia is a cause of unconsciousness before the onset of hepatic encephalopathy
B. The early finding of a low pH is a more significant risk factor than the finding of a raised pH
C. Prothrombin time greater than 60 s is an indication for liver transplantation
D. H2 receptor antagonists have been proved to reduce the incidence of gastrointestinal haemorrhage
E. Death is commonly due to cerebral oedema

Q5.72 A patient aged 76 is well but on routine blood test is found to have a bilirubin of 20 μmol/l, ALT of 120 IU/l, alk. phos. and albumin normal, globulin 40 g/dl and smooth muscle antibody positive 1/40, others negative. Hepatitis markers were negative and iron studies negative.

A. A liver biopsy is necessary to advise on further management
B. It is likely that treatment will be needed with prednisolone
C. The patient is at risk from bleeding from oesophageal varices
D. She should be advised that she must have no alcohol at all
E. 'Routine' liver function tests are a bad idea

Q5.73 Hypoxia in chronic liver disease may be caused by:

A. Pancreatic shunting
B. Intra-pulmonary shunting
C. Splinting of the diaphragm
D. Polycythaemia
E. Intracerebral shunting

Q5.74 A 25-year-old female was thrown from a horse and required emergency surgery with splenectomy. Clear fluid approximately 100 ml per day leaked from the wound and was collected in a drainage bag:

A. Fluid will burn the skin on day one of the fluid leakage
B. The serum amylase will be raised to 1000 IU
C. The fluid will have a high bicarbonate 113 meq/l
D. Enteropeptidase is present in the subcutaneous tissues
E. Octreotide can be helpful in the management

Q5.75 Following right hepatic lobe resection:

A. The liver undergoes hypertrophy
B. The portal venous pressure will be higher than 12 mmHg
C. Hyperglycaemia may be a problem
D. The proportion of hepatic artery blood supply to portal supply will increase
E. Positive pressure ventilation will reduce hepatic venous drainage

Q5.76 In chronic liver failure:

A. Rifaximin is as effective as neomycin in the treatment of encephalopathy
B. Low zinc levels may contribute to the development of encephalopathy
C. Branched-chain amino acids are widely accepted as efficacious treatment
D. Iatrogenic factors are unlikely to account for the development of hepatic encephalopathy
E. Ten litres or more of ascites may be safely drained from the abdomen over a short period providing adequate plasma expansion is achieved

Q5.77 The following statements are true about γ-glutamyl transferase (GT):

A. GT occurs mainly in the liver, kidney, pancreas and prostate
B. Plasma GT activity is higher in women than in men
C. In pregnancy plasma GT levels do not increase
D. A patient can be labelled alcoholic on the basis of an elevated GT level alone
E. GT is a sensitive indicator of liver damage

Q5.78 Reye's syndrome in children causes:

A. Acute fatty infiltration of the liver
B. Severe metabolic alkalosis
C. High plasma transaminase levels
D. Severe hyperbilirubinaemia
E. Raised plasma α-fetoprotein levels

Q5.79 Disappearing bile ducts on liver histology can occur in the following conditions:

A. Chronic autoimmune hepatitis
B. Primary biliary cirrhosis
C. Primary sclerosing cholangitis
D. Alcoholic liver disease
E. Liver transplant rejection

Q5.80 Unconjugated hyperbilirubinaemia occurs in the following familial conditions:

A. Gilbert's syndrome
B. Crigler–Najjar syndrome
C. Dubin–Johnson syndrome
D. Rotor syndrome
E. Primary hyperbilirubinaemia

5. Answers

A5.1
A. True
B. True
C. True
D. True
E. True

The principal means of transmission are via blood and blood products. HCV infection is characteristically a chronic but progressive problem which may lead to severe liver damage. He could have combined viral and alcoholic liver problems. Specific therapy is unlikely to be helpful though avoidance of alcohol may be.

A5.2
A. True
B. False
C. True
D. True
E. True

The principal plane (Cantlie's) line which divides the liver into two halves with separate biliary drainage, portal venous and hepatic arterial supply separates segments I, II, III and IV from V, VI, VII and VIII. It is an oblique plane which runs antero-posteriorly from the medial margin of the gallbladder bed to the vena cava. The portal vein carries approximately 75% of the blood supply to the liver. The left lobe of the liver consists of a medial sector (segments I and IV) lying to the right of the ligamentum teres and a lateral sector (segments II and III) to the left of the ligamentum teres.

A5.3
A. False
B. False
C. True
D. False
E. True

Stigmata of chronic liver disease suggest an intrahepatic cause of the jaundice

A5.4

A. False
B. True
C. True
D. False
E. False

Ascites accumulates because of a reduced excretion of sodium, which can be treated by reducing sodium intake. Water excretion may also be reduced leading to a fall in plasma sodium concentration. This should be treated by reducing fluid intake. Where diuretics are used, a loss of one litre daily (1 kg body weight/day) is optimal as this approximates to the maximum rate at which fluid can move from the extravascular ascites into the intravascular compartment.

A5.5

A. True
B. False
C. False
D. True
E. False

Alcohol consumption has actually fallen in France and the USA, probably because of health campaigning. However, actual intake is much greater in France, Spain, Italy and Germany than in the UK, possibly because of their well developed wine industries. Women are drinking more and seem to be more susceptible to liver damage.

A5.6

A. False
B. True
C. True
D. True
E. True

None of these signs are totally specific but provide important clues. By contrast Campbell de Morgan spots have no more significance than freckles or red hair.

A5.7

A. False
B. True
C. True
D. False
E. True

This should not be a risk with modern anti-hypertensive drugs. Methyldopa may also cause jaundice because of haemolytic anaemia. Many of the antituberculous drugs can cause liver damage, but not ethambutol or strepto-mycin. The anti-muscle spasm agent dantrolene is linked with hepato-toxicity.

A5.8
A. False
B. False
C. True
D. False
E. True
The majority of patients fail to clear the virus after an initial infection, which is usually asymptomatic. Progress to more severe liver disease may be related to the viral load, which is greater in post-transfusion patients. Although interferon suppresses viral replication in a significant proportion of patients, permanent elimination occurs only in a minority.

A5.9
A. False
B. True
C. True
D. False
E. False
Veno-occlusive disease may be caused by bush tea and homeopathic remedies. Secondary biliary cirrhosis can occur with biliary obstruction or common bile duct stones. Cirrhosis is not usually seen with metabolic disorders of glycogen metabolism even when the liver is affected.

A5.10
A. False
B. True
C. True
D. True
E. False
Liver abscess is often linked with portal vein pyaemia, but ascending cholangitis is a more usual cause. Amoebic abscess responds well to metronidazole and drainage is not usually required.

A5.11
A. False
B. True
C. False
D. True
E. True

The most likely cause is primary sclerosing cholangitis. Cholangiography will be abnormal with strictures and dilatation and liver histology is characteristic as well. There is a strong but not specific association with pANCA. Mitochondrial antibody is linked to primary biliary cirrhosis, where jaundice is late and permanent, and pain is not a prominent feature. Primary sclerosing cholangitis is frequently co-existent with ulcerative colitis.

A5.12
A. False
B. True
C. True
D. True
E. True

Hepatitis A never causes chronic liver problems. Alcohol causes cirrhosis before hepatoma, but aflatoxin from *Aspergillus flavus* is a direct carcinogen.

A5.13
A. True
B. True
C. True
D. True
E. True

Though cirrhosis is often present this is not always the case and all these conditions can cause ascites and variceal bleeding. Sometimes no cause can be found.

A5.14
A. True
B. True
C. True
D. False
E. True

Adverse hepatic reactions to penicillin are rare. Disturbed 'liver function' tests are a feature of many infections, but not usually so pronounced. Chronic autoimmune hepatitis might be a background illness predisposing to lower respiratory tract infection.

A5.15
A. True
B. True
C. True
D. True
E. True

Haemochromatosis causes cirrhosis and hepatoma, though treatment in the early stages should protect from this. Gallstones and pancreatic carcinoma are common causes of cholestasis which may be a co-incidental finding to his other diagnosis. Itching is often helped by bile acid binding therapy, though diarrhoea can be linked with steatorrhoea resulting from bile acid deficiency in the intestine.

A5.16
A. True
B. True
C. True
D. False
E. True
Both sexual and blood transmission occur with HBV, but it does not spread by ordinary social contact. Vertical transmission from mother to children can occur, but only in the neonatal period and for some reason this is particularly common in women of Chinese extraction. The partner is at risk of infection and full protection should be offered with both immuno-globulins and vaccines. The success of immunisation should be assessed by subsequent estimation of the hepatitis B surface antibody titre. Patients with HBV are at higher risk of HIV as the route of infection is the same. This may also be true for hepatitis C virus.

A5.17
A. True
B. True
C. True
D. False
E. True
A postmenopausal woman with diabetes, liver disease, and evidence of raised iron store needs to be screened for haemochromatosis. This will require liver histology, best obtained at laparoscopy in the presence of ascites. If the diagnosis is proved then venesection is used. Family screening is required with ferritin and glucose levels and HLA typing to identify early cases who may be protected from the consequence of the disease by venesection. Haemochromatosis can cause cirrhosis and lead to hepatoma, which are potentially preventable.

A5.18
A. True
B. True
C. False
D. True
E. False

HCV is transmitted parenterally by blood and its products. Transfusion donations are all screened now, but previously infections were passed on by treatment such as Factor VIII from pooled blood. Anti-HCV antibody testing by ELISA is not specific and must be confirmed by radio-immunoblot assay (RIBA) or HCV RNA testing before diagnosis is certain.

A5.19
A. False
B. True
C. True
D. True
E. True

Blood group matching is the main criterion of compatibility. Good results can be achieved in reformed alcoholics with end stage liver disease. Long-term survival is good in parenchymal liver diseases, but less impressive in hepatoma. Primary sclerosing cholangitis can be complicated by cholangio-carcinoma, not always apparent when surgery is organised, and this limits success. Patients are likely to be on azathioprine and cyclosporin or tacrolimus indefinitely, though it may be possible to withdraw such treatment in some cases eventually.

A5.20
A. False
B. False
C. True
D. True
E. True

The hallmark of chronic autoimmune hepatitis are raised aminotransferase (ALT) and immunoglobulin G levels. Serum usually contains smooth muscle and nuclear antibodies, or sometimes alternatively liver kidney microsomal (LKM) antibodies. The drawbacks of prednisolone and azathioprine therapy are justified because medical treatment does improve the shortened survival of these patients.

A5.21
A. True
B. True
C. False
D. False
E. True

This is Wernicke's encephalopathy: alcohol induced ophthalmoplegia, nystagmus and confusion. It usually responds to abstinence and vitamin supplements, especially thiamine. Alcohol intake is usually underestimated and corroborating evidence from independent sources or repeated history taking is often required. Permanent brain damage can occur, with long-term management problems.

A5.22
A. False
B. False
C. True
D. True
E. False
In alcoholic liver disease fat deposition, large mitochondria and increased iron stores are common findings, which do not themselves carry adverse significance. Alcoholic hepatitis is a serious problem associated with a definite morbidity and mortality and treatable with a course of prednisolone. Peri-venular sclerosis is a marker indicating that progression to cirrhosis is more likely.

A5.23
A. False
B. True
C. False
D. False
E. True
Acamprosate has an effect on cerebral GABA and glutamate neurotransmission, which helps reduce craving for alcohol. Antabuse is disulfiram, which blocks alcohol metabolism and encourages abstention because of unpleasant interaction with ingested alcohol leading to a build-up of acetaldehyde. Acarbose is used in diabetes to block digestion and absorption of sucrose and starch. Abciximab is an anti-platelet antibody.

A5.24
A. True
B. True
C. False
D. True
E. False
These 'biliary' enzymes are induced by various drugs including anti-convulsants and alcohol. Viral hepatitis is usually accompanied by gross elevation of transaminase, at least in the early stages. Gilbert's syndrome leads to isolated unconjugated hyperbilirubinaemia. It is not of any great medical significance but may co-exist with other problems.

A5.25
A. True
B. True
C. False
D. True
E. False

ANA is present in about 80% of patients and SMA in 70% of patients with autoimmune CAIH. AMA is virtually diagnostic of primary biliary cirrhosis, especially if M2 antibody is positive, and is absent in chronic active hepatitis.

A5.26
A. True
B. True
C. True
D. True
E. True

This is likely to be a sexually transmitted infection and partners need to be protected by barrier contraception at least until they can be shown to be immune. Most patients will clear the infection and achieve lifelong immunity: some become carriers and some of them will remain infectious long-term.

A5.27
A. True
B. False
C. False
D. True
E. False

HAV-IgG shows immunity after past hepatitis A infection, which does not cause cirrhosis. Cirrhosis is irreversible and if liver failure persists then transplantation is the only therapy likely to make a significant curative impact. Autoimmune markers such as nuclear, smooth muscle, liver kidney microsomal and mitochondrial antibodies and anti-neutrophil cytoplasmic antibodies may be positive.

Other causes to consider are hepatitis B, haemochromatosis, Wilson's disease, α_1-antitrypsin deficiency, and drug therapy.

A5.28
A. False
B. True
C. True
D. True
E. True

If the patient has taken this amount of co-proxamol then late liver damage, respiratory depression and coma are theoretical risks. However, psychopathic behaviour is often associated with untruthful accounts and it is too long after the reported overdose of pills for acetylcysteine to be very effective unless definite liver coma supervenes. Alcohol withdrawal features may occur after two or three days abstinence, but it is unlikely that formal psychiatric care would be beneficial.

A5.29
A. True
B. True
C. True
D. True
E. True

All these diagnoses are possible. A history of possible exposure and appropriate blood tests will help with A to D. Lymphoma may be difficult to prove without node biopsy and CT scanning.

A5.30
A. False
B. True
C. False
D. True
E. False

Acute alcoholic live disease may take several forms including a marked cholestasis – as in this case. It is possible that his presentation has been precipitated by hepatitis C infection – the hepatitis precedes the appearances of detectable levels of antibody by some weeks and antibody testing should be repeated in three months time. Intercurrent infection, e.g. pneumonia, should be sought and attention should be given to nutrition. Delirium tremens is a common consequence of abrupt alcohol withdrawal and Wernicke's encephalopathy should be prevented by high dose thiamine. It is unlikely that hepatic encephalopathy will develop while the prothrombin time remains normal.

A5.31
A. False
B. True
C. True
D. False
E. True

Obstructive jaundice with anaemia and melaena would strongly suggest carcinoma of the ampulla of Vater. Carcinoma of the head of the pancreas would be an important differential diagnosis, and his smoking would be a predisposing factor. Previous Billroth I gastrectomy would increase his risks of developing gastric carcinoma with metastatic lymph nodes obstructing the bile duct. Dilated bile ducts and normal albumin would go against a diagnosis of alcoholic liver disease. Painless obstructive jaundice and anaemia would argue against a diagnosis of choledocholithiasis.

A5.32
A. False
B. True
C. False
D. False
E. False

A5.33
A. False
B. False
C. True
D. False
E. True

The antimitochondrial antibody (AMA) is directed against a number of mitochondrial autoantigens including the pyruvate dehydrogenase complex. The titre of AMA does not correlate with histological stages or prognosis. Destruction of the bile ducts is mediated by T-lymphocytes. Colchicine may improve the biochemical features of cholestasis, but not the histology. Renal tubular acidosis is well recognised in primary biliary cirrhosis.

A5.34
A. False
B. False
C. True
D. False
E. False

A5..35
A. False
B. False
C. True
D. False
E. False

Wilson's disease is often associated with a low level of caeruloplasmin, but plasma levels may be normal in up to 20% of patients. Wilson's disease is thought to be caused by a defect in the gene which codes for a liver-specific copper transporting ATPase. Neurological presentation is very rare under the age of 10 years. Acute haemolytic anaemia may be a presenting feature, thought to be caused by toxic effects of copper on red blood cells. Raised 24 hour urinary copper excretion may occur in other liver diseases such as chronic active hepatitis. The most useful screening test for Wilson's disease is to repeat the 24 hour urinary copper measurement after a challenge with penicillamine, when a significant rise in the urinary copper excretion is seen. Penicillamine chelation therapy is the treatment of choice; trientine is the second line therapy for patients unable to tolerate penicillamine.

A5.36
A. False
B. False
C. True
D. True
E. False

A5.37
A. False
B. False
C. True
D. False
E. False

A5.38
A. False
B. True
C. False
D. True
E. False

Ursodeoxycholic acid will dissolve small radiolucent gallstones in about two-thirds of patients. It is the only standard specific treatment for primary biliary cirrhosis. It has been proposed for many other purposes but is not yet established: it may have a role in primary sclerosing cholangitis, chronic autoimmune hepatitis, and benign intra-hepatic cholestasis of pregnancy.

A5.39
A. True
B. True
C. True
D. True
E. True

Proliferating malignant cells recapitulate some of the phenotypic characteristic of developing foetal tissues. α-Fetoprotein can be depressed under conditions of sudden irregular hepatic cell replication as in hepato-cellular carcinoma.

A5.40
A. True
B. False
C. False
D. True
E. True

Nitrates and beta blockers are both portal hypotensive agents. To date beta blockers alone have been shown to reduce both incidence and mortality of acute variceal bleeding.

A5.41
A. False
B. True
C. False
D. True
E. True

A5.42
A. False
B. False
C. True
D. True
E. False

N-Acetylcysteine protects against liver damage by production of cysteine which acts as a glutathione donor. It also acts by supplying additional thiol groups to bind directly with the active metabolite, i.e. it scavenges the toxic metabolite and encourages its reduction to paracetamol but does not reduce the production of *N*-acetyl-*p*-benzoquinoneimine. 20–30% of *N*-acetyl-cysteine is renally excreted. The remainder undergoes first pass metabolism in the gut and liver.

A5.43
A. True
B. True
C. True
D. True
E. True

Hepatic damage is thought to be a 'group effect' of non-steroidal drugs and can occur at any time after a drug administration, though is commonest within a few weeks of initiation of therapy. Risk factors include female sex, age over 50, and underlying autoimmune disease, though whether this merely reflects the population ingesting non-steroidals remains unclear. Two discrete patterns of injury occur. One shows serological and histological features of autoimmune chronic hepatitis and the other an acute hepatitis with significantly elevated transaminase and sometimes eosinophilia.

A5.44
A. True
B. True
C. True
D. True
E. True

A5.45
A. False
B. True
C. False
D. True
E. False

A5.46
A. False
B. True
C. False
D. True
E. False

In CAIH steroids are necessary to induce remission though azathioprine is widely used as steroid sparing agent and can be used to maintain remission after steroids have been withdrawn. The timing of discontinuation of treatment remains controversial but is generally not recommended before two years and probably five years is better. After withdrawal of therapy the risk of relapse is high and long-term intensive monitoring is essential. Early reports of an association with HCV have not been confirmed, though a strong association with type II CAIH persists.

A5.47
A. False
B. False
C. True
D. False
E. False

In hereditary haemochromatosis removal of the excess iron normalises the life expectancy and the risk of HCC development in non-cirrhotic patients but in cirrhotic patients these remain higher than predicted. Cardiac dysfunction due to a dilated cardiomyopathy is a frequent complication of haemochromatosis. Treatment is with venesection except where there is haemodynamic instability since much more iron is removed by venesection. Excessive beer drinking is thought to be an aetiological factor in sub-Saharan iron overload which has different genetic abnormalities to hereditary haemochromatosis.

A5.48
A. True
B. True
C. False
D. True
E. False

A5.49
A. False
B. True
C. False
D. False
E. False

The major prognostic features in a patient with paracetamol-induced hepatotoxicity are the degree of encephalopathy, prothrombin time and renal function. Transaminases and bilirubin are not helpful. An arterial acidosis (pH < 7.30) which does not respond to fluids predicts an 80-90% mortality without transplant, and arterial pH measurement should be performed promptly where there is significant paracetamol hepatotoxicity to identify these patients. Advice should be sought from a local Liver Unit. N-Acetylcysteine improves outcome (by reducing renal and cardiovascular failure) and its use by continuous infusion until liver synthetic function recovers is now standard. Hypotension is common in acute liver failure and central line monitoring with a CVP or Swan–Ganz catheter is necessary to gauge the requirement for fluids or inotropes. The internal jugular is much safer than the sub-clavian approach in the presence of coagulopathy.

A5.50
A. True
B. False
C. True
D. False
E. False

Most cases of primary HCC arise in cirrhotic liver, irrespective of aetiology. PBC has a much smaller risk of HCC development than predicted. The HBV genome very rarely causes HCC by site-specific activation of cellular oncogenes but contains non-specific transcriptional transactivator genes which are directly oncogenic. HCV is strongly associated with HCC development though the mechanism is not known since no other RNA virus, including flaviviral special, is associated with oncogenicity.

A5.51
A. False
B. False
C. False
D. False
E. False
Interferon-α 3 million units three times weekly for six months is indicated in hepatitis B carriers where hepatitis B e antigen is present and infectivity and virulence are high. Therapy is aimed at converting from hepatitis B e antigen to hepatitis B e antibody positivity. It is also useful in hepatitis C when 3 million to 6 million units three times weekly for 6–12 months is used. It is also used in hairy cell leukaemia but has no role in acute hepatitis.

A5.52
A. True
B. False
C. True
D. False
E. False
After cholecystectomy stones may form in the common bile duct even after many years. Common duct stones, unlike gallbladder stones, are not reliably detected by ultrasonography. The unobstructed common duct may measure up to 10 mm post-cholecystectomy. Jaundice following treatment with co-amoxiclav (amoxycillin/clavulanic acid) is an increasingly recognised drug reaction and may be delayed up to 2 months after drug exposure.

A5.53
A. False
B. False
C. False
D. False
E. False
Genetic studies have shown that most families have different mutations in the gene and, therefore, screening is not possible. The genetic defect is useful only within family studies. The gene responsible is a p-type ATPase thought to be involved in copper transport and the low caeruloplasmin levels found in Wilson's disease are an epiphenomenon. A high urinary copper excretion is suggestive of Wilson's disease but is also found in

some acute hepatitides, e.g. acute hepatitis A. Zinc is thought to be a safe treatment and is used as second line maintenance therapy. Stopping treatment leads to a rapid deterioration which is often fatal, thought to be due to release of copper from non-toxic stores.

A5.54
A. True
B. True
C. True
D. True
E. False

The use of TIPSS as an alternative to surgery has been successfully used for the treatment of recurrent and acute variceal haemorrhage and is now well established. Its actions are identical to previously used surgical shunt procedures varying only in the size of the shunt. Acute liver failure is well recognised and may be due to diversion of portal blood with its supply of growth factors. The major complication is that of new or worsening hepatic encephalopathy.

A5.55
A. False
B. True
C. True
D. False
E. True

Treatment is targeted at treating the underlying cause and reducing gut protein and bacterial overload.

A5.56
A. False
B. True
C. True
D. False
E. True

A5.57
A. True
B. True
C. False
D. False
E. True

A5.58
A. True
B. True
C. False
D. True
E. False

Disappearing bile ducts and granulomas are histological features of primary biliary cirrhosis.

A5.59
A. False
B. False
C. False
D. False
E. True

This lady had focal microvesicular steatosis secondary to HRT. She is a good example of why it is important to obtain histology to 'prove' the diagnosis of cancer.

A5.60
A. False
B. False
C. False
D. True
E. False

Unfortunately LFTs in chronic hepatitis C virus infection give no reliable indication to activity or infectivity, but positive hepatitis C RNA by PCR indicates continued viral presence. Interferon-α is licensed for the treatment of hepatitis C virus infection although only 25% of cases demonstrate any sustained response to treatment. Vertical transmission from mother to baby occurs in < 10%. Parenteral transmission (i.v. drug abuse/blood product transfusion) is the commonest mode of infection. Hepatitis C virus infection in the absence of significant liver disease does not significantly affect fetal viability.

A5.61
A. False
B. False
C. True
D. True
E. True

Most patients will require lifelong immune-suppression with drugs like azathioprine and cyclosporin. However, it may be possible to withdraw them altogether eventually in some patients. Prednisolone is used in the early phase and tailed off. High dose steroids and subsequent tacrolimus therapy are used after rejection episodes.

Levamisole is not used – it is an immune stimulant.

A5.62

A. True
B. True
C. True
D. False
E. True

Blood alcohol is a marker of recent alcohol abuse. Serum bilirubin can be raised in a variety of diseases and can, therefore, not be used as a marker. CDT and MCV are useful markers for alcohol abuse rather than alcoholic liver damage.

A5.63

A. False
B. False
C. True
D. False
E. True

A5.64

A. True
B. True
C. True
D. False
E. False

Large duct obstruction is excluded by normal ERCP. Carbon tetrachloride poisoning is rare and gives rise to toxic hepatitis rather than cholestasis.

A percutaneous liver biopsy should give helpful information. This could be chronic autoimmune hepatitis, primary biliary cirrhosis, alcoholic liver disease or drug toxicity. Patients often forget to mention the use of sex steroids, and they may conceal their true alcohol intake. A course of glucocorticoids with or without cholestyramine should help resolve the symptoms.

A5.65

A. True
B. False
C. True
D. True
E. False

Chronic viral hepatitis accounts for around 30% of all graft recipients world-wide and is the single commonest indication for transplantation. Many centres restrict grafting to those without detectable HBV DNA. Viral recurrence is very common for both hepatitis B and C viruses, probably as a result of extrahepatic sites of replication. In hepatitis B, viral load predicts outcome, and in those with detectable HBV DNA, polyclonal human HB specific Ig improves graft survival. No such immunoglobulin is available for HCV, where although viral recurrence is almost universal disease recurrence is slower and more indolent than for HBV. In HCV overall survival is 87–100% at 2 years, but there is 50% disease recurrence at 5 years. Fibrosing cholestatic hepatitis occurs in the context of immuno-suppression and chronic hepatitis B, and is characterised by rapidly progressive hepatic failure, periportal fibrosis with intense cholestasis but no cirrhosis, mild inflammatory cellular infiltrate, and high expression of B viral antigens from the hepatocytes.

A5.66
A. False
B. True
C. True
D. False
E. False

Hepatitis A only affects individuals once, and IgM antibody is character-istic of current or very recent infection. IgG antibody can occur early, but then persists long-term. It reflects exposure (which may be inapparent especially in children), and immunity to reinfection. Hepatitis A is an acute illness with jaundice and gastroenteritis. It rarely progresses to liver failure and never becomes chronic.

A5.67
A. False
B. True
C. False
D. False
E. True

A5.68
A. True
B. False
C. True
D. False
E. True

Hepatic encephalopathy (coma) may occur in liver failure from any cause. GI haemorrhage is a potent precipitant largely due to the protein load delivered to the bowel. All sedative drugs carry the risk of precipitating hepatic encephalopathy but particularly the benzo-diazepines and drugs acting on opiate receptors. The synthetic disaccharide lactulose NOT lactose is used in the treatment of hepatic encephalopathy

A5.69
A. False
B. True
C. False
D. False
E. False

The first most useful investigation would be ultrasonography to search for biliary tree obstruction. Liver biopsy is contra-indicated in patients with marked biliary obstruction (which this patient may have), and also in patients with gross ascites, as it carries a lower success rate with increased complications. Laparoscopy permits direct visualisation of the liver surface and peritoneum, and (targeted) safer liver biopsy. Wilson's disease is vanishingly rare presenting over the age of 50 years. Diuretic therapy, gross ascites itself, and prolonged hospital stays have significant complication rates: therapeutic paracentesis is safe when carried out with appropriate plasma expansion. Variceal eradication by banding or sclerotherapy is indicated only in patients who have had an index variceal bleed. Studies have not demonstrated any benefit in non-bleeders, in whom propranolol has been shown to reduce bleeding rates.

A5.70
A. True
B. False
C. True
D. False
E. False

Liver disease secondary to heart failure is common. The liver derives most of its oxygen second hand after the intestine has had its share and so congestive cardiac failure with raised hepatic (not portal) vein pressure and reduced cardiac output will result in abnormal liver function tests and sometimes hepatic encephalopathy. The cause of weight loss is not clear but is seldom the result of steatorrhoea.

A5.71
A. True
B. False
C. False
D. True
E. True

Early alkalosis is a significant risk factor and one would watch for hypoglycaemia before the onset of hepatic encephalopathy. A prothrombin time greater than 100s is the normal trigger for transplantation. H2 receptor antagonists have been shown in a controlled trial to reduce the instance of GI haemorrhage.

A5.72
A. False
B. False
C. False
D. False
E. True

Most physicians would think the risk of liver biopsy (one death per thousand) would not justify this in an asymptomatic patient with only mildly abnormal 'liver function' tests. The 'liver function' tests should be monitored. There is no evidence that the occasional drink will make any difference, and, if she were to enjoy a drinks holiday, might reduce her quality of life. There should always be a reason for doing tests, in the patient's own interests.

A5.73
A. False
B. True
C. True
D. True
E. False

Intra-pulmonary shunting ('spider naevi in the lungs'), splinting of the diaphragms and polycythaemia may all contribute to hypoxia in chronic liver disease.

A5.74
A. False
B. False
C. True
D. False
E. True

Pancreatic juice is very alkaline compared with plasma. Endopeptidase is found in the intestinal brush border of the upper small bowel and activates trypsinogen to trypsin. The juice only causes redness of subcutaneous tissue and skin after a couple of days because of the alkaline nature, not because of the activated pancreatic fistula fluid.

A5.75
A. True
B. False
C. False
D. False
E. True

The liver contains about 100 000 acini and the remaining acini after resection grow larger. The ratio of the hepatic artery blood (1:3) to portal blood (2:3) remains relatively constant for normal liver tissue. Care of the patient in the postoperative period must include careful monitoring for hypoglycaemia, for hypokalaemia, and hypoalbuminaemia, which may affect renal functions. Normal breathing creates negative intrathoracic pressure which aids venous drainage from the inferior vena cava.

A5.76
A. True
B. True
C. False
D. False
E. True

In hepatic failure encephalopathy is precipitated by several factors including gastrointestinal bleeding, constipation, spontaneous bacterial peritonitis, non-compliance with drugs or protein restriction, sedative drugs and diuretics, alcohol and development of a hepatocellular carcinoma. Osmotic laxatives relieve constipation and purge dietary and epithelial sources of ammonia, while non-absorbed antibiotics reduce the ammonia-forming bacteria in the gut. When neomycin is contraindicated (e.g. due to renal failure) rifaximin or metronidazole are equally effective. Two of the five enzymes which convert ammonia into urea are zinc-dependent and zinc levels should be checked. Branched-chain amino acids theoretically reduce the availability of aromatic amino acids to act as false neuro-transmitters, but clinical results are equivocal and use is not widespread. Paracentesis carries the risks of introducing sepsis and vascular or bowel injury, but the risk of causing circulatory collapse by rapid fluid shifts is effectively prevented by giving plasma expanders such as 20% albumin solution or dextrans, and this procedure is safe in refractory ascites.

A5.77
A. True
B. False
C. True
D. False
E. True

Plasma GT activity is higher in men than women. Drugs like pheno-barbitone, phenytoin and alcohol can induce GT synthesis without cell damage. Moderately raised levels of GT (up to about three times the reference limit) are particularly difficult to interpret.

A5.78
A. True
B. False
C. True
D. False
E. False

Reye's syndrome causes marked encephalopathy in children. It is associated with severe hypoglycaemia, severe metabolic acidosis and only mild elevation in plasma bilirubin. The aetiology is uncertain but there seems to be an association with aspirin ingestion.

A5.79
A. False
B. True
C. True
D. False
E. True

Ductopenic liver transplant rejection is a serious condition not reversible by immunosuppression and usually needing retransplantation. The onset is from 6 weeks to 9 months post-transplant, but usually within 3 months. Primary biliary cirrhosis and primary sclerosing cholangitis are the other two conditions where ductular damage occurs.

A5.80
A. True
B. True
C. False
D. False
E. True

Gilbert's syndrome presents with a rise in unconjugated bilirubin because of defects in bilirubin metabolism and also its excretion. Crigler–Najjar syndrome has deficiency in conjugation enzyme causing severe unconjugated hyperbilirubinaemia. Primary hyperbilirubinaemia is a rare condition caused by premature destruction of abnormal red cell precursors and haemolysis.

6. Pancreas, Biliary System, Peritoneum and General

Q6.1 **At endoscopic retrograde cholangiopancreatography (ERCP) the pancreatic duct is:**

A. Always demonstrated
B. Sharply cut off or strictured in carcinoma
C. Irregular with dilated side branches in acute pancreatitis
D. Normal in non-insulin dependent diabetes mellitus
E. Usually positioned obliquely across the mid line

Q6.2 **A young Irish female smoker presents with muscle weakness, limb discomfort and long-standing diarrhoea. Her potassium is normal. Alkaline phosphatase was elevated. Barium follow-through is normal. What blood tests would prove particularly useful:**

A. Alpha 1 glycoprotein
B. Calcium level
C. Alanine aminotransferase (ALT)
D. Anti-endomysial antibody
E. Anti-cholinesterase inhibitor antibody

Q6.3 **Treatment of gallstones might include:**

A. Laparoscopic cholecystectomy
B. External shock-wave lithotripsy
C. Octreotide
D. Drastic weight reduction
E. Ursodeoxycholic acid

Q6.4 **A 45-year-old woman with a history of by-pass surgery for unresectable pancreatic carcinoma presents with fever, painful jaundice and anaemia. The following are likely:**

A. Biliary obstruction from recurrent tumour
B. Ascending cholangitis
C. Diffuse intravascular coagulation
D. Chronic pancreatitis
E. Liver abscess

Q6.5   The frequency of gallstones in developed countries:

A. Can be measured by population ultrasonography survey
B. Closely relates to cholecystectomy rates
C. Is increasing
D. May be estimated from review of autopsies
E. Correlates strongly with age

Q6.6   Elevation of carbohydrate antigen CA19-9 is seen in pancreatic carcinoma. It is not completely specific and may also occur in:

A. Gallstones
B. Cholangiocarcinoma
C. Gilbert's syndrome
D. Hepatitis
E. Hepatoma

Q6.7   At ERCP a sharply defined cut-off is noted in the common hepatic duct with no contrast entering the right and left hepatic ducts. This is consistent with:

A. Carcinoma of the head of the pancreas
B. Primary sclerosing cholangitis
C. Metastatic carcinoma in local lymph nodes
D. Cholangiocarcinoma
E. Cholelithiasis

Q6.8   A 47-year-old woman had a history of aorto-iliac thrombosis 9 years before. She had been on the oral contraceptive pill and had been sterilised two months prior to this event. Serum cholesterol was 8 mmol/l and she smoked cigarettes. She attended clinic with a one-year history of alternating diarrhoea and constipation 2–3 times weekly. There was no rectal bleeding and her weight was steady. The diagnoses to consider are:

A. Irritable bowel syndrome
B. Ulcerative colitis
C. Crohn's disease
D. Ischaemic colitis
E. Carcinoma colon

Q6.9   Primary sclerosing cholangitis:

A. Is primarily a disease of the extrahepatic bile ducts
B. Is generally associated with severe ulcerative colitis
C. Is cured by total colectomy
D. Is a risk factor for development of colon cancer complicating ulcerative colitis
E. Is mainly a disease of young females

Q6.10 Pancreatic pseudocyst:

A. Complicates chronic pancreatitis
B. Communicates with the pancreatic ductal system
C. May spontaneously resolve
D. Predisposes to pancreatic carcinoma
E. Causes increased serum lipase concentrations

Q6.11 In pancreatic failure:

A. Serum folate is typically low
B. The T:K ratio of the pancreolauryl test exceeds 40
C. Faecal fat excretion exceeds 18 mmol/day
D. Thiamine levels are reduced
E. A raised alkaline phosphatase suggests osteoporosis

Q6.12 Laparoscopic surgery:

A. Has meant the virtual demise of open cholecystectomy
B. Is feasible for nearly all abdominal surgery, including Whipple's operation
C. Has significantly shortened operating times
D. Permits discharge as early as 24 hours after cholecystectomy
E. Facilitates resection of adhesions from previous surgery

Q6.13 Severe abdominal infection may be treated with which of the following parenteral antibiotics with few side-effects:

A. Cephalexin
B. Cefuroxime
C. Cefoxitin
D. Ceftriaxone
E. Ceftazidime

Q6.14 Chronic pancreatitis:

A. Usually results from repeated attacks of acute pancreatitis
B. Is not likely to be the cause of steatorrhoea in the absence of abdominal pain
C. Is suggested by a pancreatic function test in which there is a reduced concentration of bicarbonate in a normal volume of secretion after stimulation with secretin-pancreozymin
D. Is a cause of elevated hepatic alkaline phosphatase concentration in serum
E. Is a feature of cystic fibrosis disease

Q6.15 Bile duct stones:

A. Invariably originate from the gallbladder
B. Predispose to cholangiocarcinoma
C. Can be dissolved by solvents such as methyl-tertiary-butyl-ether which are directly infused into the bile duct
D. Usually have greater than 90% cholesterol content
E. Complicate Caroli's disease

Q6.16 The following are carcinogenic in the gastrointestinal system:

A. *Clonorchis sinensis*
B. Thorotrast
C. Gastric reflux
D. Margarine yellow
E. Toluidine blue

Q6.17 The following are hamartomas of the gastrointestinal system or liver:

A. von Meyerburg complex
B. Peutz–Jeghers' syndrome
C. Brunneroma
D. Benign lymphoid polyp
E. Hyerplastic polyp

Q6.18 Pancreatitis:

A. May be caused by tumour
B. Can be caused by hypocalcaemia
C. May be caused by mumps and influenza
D. Chronic pancreatitis causes exocrine insufficiency
E. Pain will classically refer to the right shoulder tip

Q6.19 GI complications in patients with long-standing diabetes:

A. Can be reliably controlled by improving diabetic control
B. Include intractable diarrhoea
C. Respond well to prokinetic medication
D. May respond to treatment with antibiotics
E. Can give rise to a succussion splash

Q6.20 Smoking decreases the risk of developing:

A. Ulcerative colitis
B. Parkinson's disease
C. Crohn's disease
D. Alzheimer's disease
E. Motor neurone disease

Q6.21 Arthropathy is a recognised feature of:

A. Crohn's disease
B. Ulcerative colitis
C. Primary biliary cirrhosis
D. Haemochromatosis
E. Coeliac disease

Q6.22 Conformal radiotherapy:

A. Allows greater dosage to malignant tissue
B. Is an alternative name for conventional treatment
C. Depends on three-dimensional imaging techniques
D. Protects normal tissue
E. Describes obsolete treatments

Q6.23 The complications of ERCP and sphincterotomy include:

A. Cholangitis
B. Pancreatitis
C. Bleeding
D. Perforation
E. Death

Q6.24 Cholangiocarcinoma:

A. Can be distinguished from a benign biliary stricture by ERCP appearances
B. Complicates ulcerative colitis
C. Complicates primary sclerosing cholangitis
D. Is rapidly progressive, with few patients surviving longer than 3 months after diagnosis
E. Complicates liver fluke infestation

Q6.25 The following are generally accepted as being associated:

A. Gallstones and chronic pancreatitis
B. Type IIa hyperlipidaemia and chronic pancreatitis
C. Type V hyperlipidaemia and acute pancreatitis
D. Pseudocyst formation and chronic pancreatitis
E. Alcohol intake and chronic pancreatitis

Q6.26 An 18-year-old woman with cystic fibrosis who is taking high doses of pancreatic enzyme supplements presents with abdominal pain, constipation and a mass in the right iliac fossa:

A. Distal intestinal obstruction syndrome is the most likely diagnosis
B. Her dose of pancreatic enzyme supplements should be increased
C. Large doses of laxatives should be given
D. A Gastrograffin enema should be the first investigation
E. Balanced electrolyte lavage solution may be used to treat distal intestinal obstruction

Q6.27 Choledochal cyst:

A. Causes an abdominal mass
B. Predisposes to pancreatic cancer
C. Is associated with an anomalous connection between the pancreas and biliary tree
D. May involve the intrahepatic biliary tree
E. Is commoner in males

Q6.28 Drugs with very significant gastrointestinal side-effects include:

A. Clofibrate
B. Azathioprine
C. Atenolol
D. Alendronate
E. Gentamicin

Q6.29 Gallstones can be caused by:

A. Haemolytic anaemia
B. Ceftriaxone
C. Clofibrate
D. Chenodeoxycholic acid
E. Obesity

Q6.30 In metastatic disease of the liver, tumour markers indicating a pancreatic primary site include:

A. Interleukin 8 (IL-8)
B. Carcino-embryonic antigen (CEA)
C. Alpha fetoprotein (AFP)
D. Carbohydrate antigen 125 (CA-125)
E. Carbohydrate antigen 19-9 (CA 19-9)

Q6.31 A 65-year-old male presented with severe upper abdominal pain and vomiting. A diagnosis of severe pancreatitis was made on the basis of a blood pH of 7.2, pO_2 8 KP, serum amylase 1350 iu/l, aspartate transaminase 175 iu/l, blood glucose 11.2 mmol/l and serum calcium 1.89 iu/l:

A. Early ultrasound and CT scanning should be undertaken to monitor the development of any complication
B. Even in the presence of progressive jaundice an ERCP should not be performed in the first six weeks
C. Early oral feeding is of benefit
D. Pethidine can be used as an analgesic
E. Early surgery will reduce morbidity

Q6.32 Which of the following features are common in steatorrhoea caused by pancreatic exocrine insufficiency:

A. A diabetic glucose tolerance curve
B. Oil droplets in the faeces
C. Recurrent attacks of severe upper abdominal pain
D. Cholelithiasis
E. The steatorrhoea is cured by giving sodium bicarbonate

Q6.33 Investigation of the pancreaticobiliary tree by endoscopic retrograde cholangiopancreatography (ERCP):

A. Is not possible in patients who have had a Polya gastrectomy
B. Is useful in the diagnosis of primary sclerosing cholangitis
C. May cause pancreatitis
D. Requires a general anaesthetic
E. Is contraindicated in extrahepatic biliary obstruction because of the risk of developing hepatorenal failure

Q6.34 In a patient presenting with ascites:

A. Spontaneous bacterial peritonitis is indicated by an ascitic neutrophil count in excess of 250/mm^3
B. Pancreatic carcinoma is excluded if the ascites is chylous
C. Who has chronic liver disease and a serum sodium of 129 mmol/l, treatment with normal saline is required
D. If secondary to chronic liver disease diuretics are appropriate first-line treatment
E. The finding of spider naevi indicates alcoholic liver disease

Q6.35 The following drugs cause gastrointestinal side-effects that are often seen in clinical practice:

A. Mefenamic acid
B. Fluoxetine
C. Aspirin
D. Mesalazine
E. Sulphasalazine

Q6.36 A 45-year-old man with weight loss, diarrhoea and recent onset of diabetes mellitus is referred for investigation and found to have diffuse pancreatic calcification:

A. This is only found in neuroendocrine tumours of the pancreas producing a parathormone-like substance
B. The development of diabetes mellitus indicates an autoimmune cause
C. An alcohol history is important
D. Xylose absorption studies are likely to be normal
E. Treatment of the diabetes will reverse the calcification

Q6.37 The stimuli for release of secretin are:

A. Acid in the duodenum
B. Stimulation of vagus nerve
C. Site or smell of food
D. Hypoglycaemia
E. Somatostatin release

Q6.38 A 25-year-old violent institutionalised schizophrenic patient developed high swinging pyrexia. Chest x-ray and abdominal x-ray showed a large gas bubble in the right hypochondrium. Laparoscopy under general anaesthetic revealed a subphrenic abscess which was cleared with suction. Endoscopy under the same anaesthetic revealed a large duodenal ulcer. Post-operatively the chest x-ray showed the same gas bubble unchanged in size:

A. Perforation of the duodenal ulcer is the most likely cause of the gas bubble
B. Pus in the abdomen can pass into the chest
C. Lung abscess can penetrate into the abdomen
D. The duodenal ulcer can cause the lung abscess
E. Psychiatric drug therapy may suppress GI symptoms

Q6.39 In acute pancreatitis the following are clinical features of a more severe disease:

A. Blood glucose < 10 mmol/l
B. Serum calcium < 2.0 mmol/l
C. White blood cell count < $15 \times 10^9/l$
D. Serum urea < 16 mmol/l
E. Arterial oxygen saturation (PaO_2) < 60 mmol/l

Q6.40 The following conditions are recognised causes of right upper quadrant pain:

A. Fatty liver
B. Acute cholecystitis
C. Alcoholic hepatitis
D. Peptic ulcer disease
E. Pancreatitis

Q6.41 Rapid onset of ascites can be explained by:

A. Acute pancreatitis
B. Ovarian carcinoma
C. Cirrhosis
D. Hepatoma
E. Portal vein thrombosis

Q6.42 Drugs of relevance to gastrointestinal function:

A. Nitrates, given for angina, may aggravate heartburn and reflux
B. Proton pump inhibitors, given for dyspepsia, may enhance the effect of mesalazine in the form of Asacol
C. Verapamil, given for hypertension, may induce constipation
D. Sulphasalazine, given for rheumatoid arthritis, may induce epigastric pain
E. Domperidone, given for nausea, may cause galactorrhoea

Q6.43 A 34-year-old man presents with a 6-month story of intermittent loose stools and gradual weight loss of about 3 kg in spite of eating normally. He has mild, iron-deficiency anaemia. He reports no abdominal pain and has not seen blood in the stools. He drinks about 30 units of alcohol per week but has taken no medication. Full colonoscopy was entirely normal.

A. 10% of patients presenting with chronic pancreatitis have not experienced pain
B. A raised platelet count could indicate Crohn's disease
C. Features of hyposplenism in the blood film would increase the likelihood of coeliac disease
D. A negative stool culture would be unusual if his problem is due to giardiasis
E. A positive test for lactose intolerance would make duodenal biopsies unnecessary

6. Answers

A6.1
A. False
B. True
C. False
D. True
E. True

The pancreatic duct is not always filled at ERCP, and indeed it may be best to avoid this where the interest is in biliary disease, since iatrogenic pancreatitis can occur after contrast injection. Chronic pancreatitis can cause distortion of the duct, but this is not generally a feature of acute pancreatitis. Diabetes is a disease of the islets and does not normally affect exocrine pancreatic function or architecture.

A6.2
A. False
B. True
C. False
D. True
E. False

The clinical picture suggests coeliac disease with osteomalacia. She had an osteomalacic myopathy and treatment with calcium and a gluten free diet rendered her symptom-free.

A6.3
A. True
B. True
C. False
D. False
E. True

The standard treatment for gallbladder stones is cholecystectomy. Disruption and dissolution of stones are alternatives used in a small minority of cases. Both the somatostatin agonist octreotide and bariatric surgery or severe dieting may actually cause gallstones.

A6.4
A. True
B. True
C. True
D. True
E. True
Any of these could be the explanation. The outlook is poor but a trial of antibiotic therapy would be useful.

A6.5
A. True
B. False
C. True
D. True
E. True
At least 70% of gallbladder stones are asymptomatic. Measuring prevalence by ultrasonography of the community or reviewing autopsy results, adding cholecystectomy to current gallstone frequency, will give reasonable estimates. There is a very poor correlation between gallstone prevalence and surgical rates, which vary widely over time and between countries.

A6.6
A. False
B. True
C. False
D. True
E. True
The presence of a markedly raised CA19-9 should always lead to consideration of carcinoma of the pancreas as a cause, but it may occur in other tumours such as bile duct and primary liver carcinomas. It may rise non-specifically in liver inflammation. A more specific test for hepatoma is α-fetoprotein.

A6.7
A. False
B. True
C. True
D. True
E. False
A high complete obstruction suggests malignancy, either a primary bile acid tumour or extrinsic pressure from nodes involved in metastases. Primary sclerosing cholangitis may cause occlusive strictures in the large ducts as well as in the liver.

Pancreatic head carcinoma would obstruct the common bile duct, and gallstones in the proximal bile ducts generally are mobile and non-obstructing.

A6.8
A. True
B. True
C. True
D. True
E. True
It is most likely that she has irritable bowel syndrome or possibly bowel ischaemia because of her past history. However, inflammatory bowel disease needs to be ruled out and can itself be associated with thrombotic disease. Any alteration of bowel habit needs to be investigated to exclude carcinoma in this age group. Thyroid over-activity also sometimes shows up in this way.

A6.9
A. False
B. False
C. False
D. True
E. False
Primary sclerosing cholangitis is characterised by an obliterative inflammatory fibrosis usually involving the whole of the biliary tree. Patients with primary sclerosing cholangitis and ulcerative colitis have a male predominance (male:female = 2:1). Though the associated ulcerative colitis (in 70% of patients with primary sclerosing cholangitis) is total in over 90% of cases, the symptoms tend to be mild, often without rectal bleeding and with prolonged remissions. Colectomy does not affect the progression of the disease. Cholangiocarcinoma may be a complication and recent evidence suggests that primary sclerosing cholangitis may be an independent risk factor for the development of dysplasia of the colon.

A6.10
A. True
B. True
C. True
D. False
E. True

A6.11
A. False
B. False
C. True
D. False
E. False

Pancreatic failure leads to reduced absorption of fat-soluble vitamins and the possibility of osteomalacia. Pancreatic lipase activity can be indirectly measured using the pancreolauryl test. Low levels are indicated by a low T/K ratio, usually less than 30.

A6.12
A. False
B. False
C. False
D. True
E. False

A6.13
A. False
B. True
C. True
D. False
E. True

Cephalosporins are potent and effective. There are few side-effects from cefuroxime and ceftazidime. Cefoxitin is a cephamycin which has a particular additional activity against obligatory anaerobes such as *Bacteroides*. These drugs should, however, be avoided in patients who have a definite significant history of penicillin allergy as there is a 10% cross re-activity. Ceftriaxone crystallises in bile and urine and can cause gallstones which may confuse diagnosis and management. Ceftazidime has enhanced activity against *Pseudomonas* and many would reserve its use where this is proven to be the pathogen. Cefixime and cephalexin are only available as oral preparations.

A6.14
A. False
B. False
C. True
D. True
E. True

A6.15
A. False
B. True
C. True
D. False
E. True

A6.16
A. True
B. True
C. True
D. False
E. False

A6.17
A. True
B. True
C. True
D. False
E. False

A6.18
A. True
B. False
C. True
D. True
E. False

A6.19
A. False
B. True
C. False
D. True
E. True

Diabetes is associated with several GI complications including gastro-paresis, bacterial overgrowth and alterations in colonic function, with autonomic neuropathy being the underlying pathological process. Gastro-paresis may give rise to a succussion splash and is sometimes responsive to prokinetic agents such as cisapride or metoclopramide, though the effects are unpredictable. Antibiotics are successful therapy for bacterial over-growth and erythromycin has been used in gastroparesis. The natural history of the various GI complications tend to be variable over time and only partially responsive to good diabetic control.

A6.20
A. True
B. True
C. False
D. True
E. False

The relationship between smoking and ulcerative colitis and Crohn's are opposite. Smokers with Crohn's disease who stop have a significantly reduced rate of relapse. Some patients with UC are worse when they stop.

A6.21
A. True
B. True
C. False
D. True
E. False

Patients with inflammatory bowel disease can have a non-erosive peripheral arthropathy associated with disease activity. They can also develop an ankylosing spondylitis and sacroiliitis unrelated to disease activity. Primary biliary cirrhosis sufferers develop arthralgia, osteoporosis and osteomalacia, but not organic joint involvement specifically. Chondro-calcinosis is a recognised feature of haemochromatosis.

A6.22
A. True
B. False
C. True
D. True
E. False

The basis of the new development of conformal radiotherapy is the acute special definition of tumour. This permits delivery of higher effective doses while sparing adjacent normal tissue. It depends on imaging by procedures such as CT and MRI scanning.

A6.23
A. True
B. True
C. True
D. True
E. True

All are true. Cholangitis occurs if contrast is injected into part of the biliary tree that is subsequently not drained, for example, above a stricture. Pancreatitis occurs in about 5% ranging from a trivial episode to a severe life-threatening illness. Perforation is rare but can occur after sphincterotomy. Bleeding occurs occasionally after sphincterotomy but can usually be controlled by adrenaline injection. The overall mortality after sphincterotomy is 0.8%.

A6.24
A. False
B. True
C. True
D. False
E. True

Cytology samples taken at ERCP result in a positive diagnosis in 75% of cases. The tumour is usually relatively slow growing with survival for up to 2 years being common, even in non-operated cases. Liver flukes (*Clonorchis sinensis*) are a cause in the Far East.

A6.25
A. False
B. False
C. True
D. True
E. True

A6.26
A. True
B. False
C. False
D. True
E. True

Distal intestinal obstruction syndrome is the most likely diagnosis, but appendix mass, Crohn's disease and fibrosing colonopathy (long segment stricture resulting from mucosal damage and fibrosis, thought to be associated with large doses of pancreatic enzyme supplements) should be considered. Gastrograffin enema is helpful in distinguishing these various conditions, and may be therapeutic in relieving the obstruction. An alternative treatment is lavage with a balanced electrolyte solution. Laxatives are usually ineffective. The dose of pancreatic enzyme supplements should not be changed until a definitive diagnosis has been made. Distal intestinal obstruction syndrome may be precipitated by inadequate enzyme supplements, but over-treatment with too large doses may increase the risk of developing fibrosing colonopathy.

A6.27
A. True
B. False
C. True
D. True
E. False

A6.28
A. True
B. True
C. False
D. True
E. False

Clofibrate (and probably all the other fibrates too) induces cholesterol gallstones, some of which become symptomatic. Alendronate increases the prevalence of oesophagitis – this may occur with other biphosphonates but this is not definite. Azapropazone is one of the more toxic non-steroidal anti-inflammatory drugs: it causes upper GI bleeding and also precipitates exacerbations in inflammatory bowel disease.

A6.29
A. True
B. True
C. True
D. False
E. True

Haemolysis leads to increases in pigment and cholesterol stones. Fibric acid derivatives work by increasing biliary cholesterol and cause cholesterol stone formation. Ceftriaxone actually crystallises in bile. Both obesity and weight reduction are associated with cholesterol stones. Bile acid therapy can dissolve cholesterol stones – ursodeoxycholic acid is generally used nowadays.

A6.30
A. False
B. False
C. False
D. True
E. True

None of the tumour markers is completely reliable. CA 19-9 is reasonably specific for pancreatic carcinoma, though sensitivity is not high. CA 125 may also be raised in this condition, but is more characteristic of ovarian carcinoma. AFP is a useful marker of primary liver cell cancer and CEA is associated with advanced and metastatic large bowel carcinoma.

A6.31

A. True
B. False
C. False
D. True
E. False

Both ultrasonography and CT scanning are important in the monitoring and assessment of severe pancreatitis to assess any fluid collections, development of cysts, necrosis or abscess. In suspected gallstone pancreatitis particularly with progressive jaundice, ERCP should be considered. Oral food intake may not be tolerated for some time and prolonged parenteral feeding may be required to maintain nutrition. Surgery is only indicated for those complications failing to resolve spontaneously as it carries a high morbidity.

A6.32

A. True
B. True
C. False
D. False
E. False

A6.33

A. False
B. True
C. True
D. False
E. False

ERCP is technically more difficult to undertake in patients who have had a Polya gastrectomy as the ampulla has to be approached from below via the afferent loop, but is not impossible. Visualisation of the extrahepatic tree is important in the diagnosis of primary sclerosing cholangitis, as liver histology is not always diagnostic. Magnetic resonance cholangiopancreatography may offer a non-invasive means of visualising the biliary tree in the future and thus avoid the risks of ERCP. Post-ERCP pancreatitis is the main cause of morbidity following diagnostic ERCP, clinically significant pancreatitis occurring in up to 3% of cases. ERCP does not normally require a general anaesthetic and can usually be performed under IV sedation. Hepatorenal failure can develop in patients with extrahepatic biliary obstruction, particularly those complicated by infection. Relief of the obstruction which can normally be achieved by endoscopic means is all important in the prevention and treatment of this complication, together with the maintenance of good hydration, and treatment of any infection.

A6.34

A. True
B. False
C. False
D. True
E. False

Spontaneous bacterial peritonitis (SBP) may complicate chronic liver disease and should be suspected in patients with worsening or resistant ascites particularly if associated with fever and/or abdominal pain although it must be noted that the classical features of peritonitis are often absent and a high index of suspicion should be practised. An elevated ascitic neutrophil count > 250/mm³ is indicative of SBP and most authorities would institute antibiotic therapy on that basis alone. Chylous ascites is due to lymphatic obstruction which may occur in pancreatic carcinoma. Hyponatraemia seen in chronic liver disease associated with ascites is *not* indicative of sodium depletion and is dilutional. Secondary hyperaldosteronism is one of the factors involved in the development of ascites. Spider naevi occur in any form of chronic liver disease and are not specific to alcoholic liver disease.

A6.35

A. True
B. True
C. True
D. False
E. True

Most of these are well recognised – perhaps not fluoxetine so much.

A6.36

A. False
B. False
C. True
D. True
E. False

Calcification commonly occurs in chronic pancreatitis, particularly of an alcoholic aetiology. Diabetes mellitus occurs in pancreatic disease from any cause if a significant amount of the gland is damaged. Xylose absorption studies are a measure of small bowel mucosal integrity. Diabetes mellitus should be treated adequately to control symptoms and prevent the complications associated with glucose intolerance but this will have no effect on pancreatic calcification.

A6.37
A. True
B. False
C. False
D. False
E. False

Vagal nerve stimulation, sight and smell of food, and hypoglycaemia may all result in pancreatic secretion but these result from stimulation of the vagus nerve not from release of secretin.

A6.38
A. False
B. True
C. False
D. True
E. True

Heavy sedation may mask a patient's abdominal pain, or pain may make psychiatric control more difficult, causing increased drug dosage. Pus in the abdomen can cause problems in the chest with effusion, empyema and fistula into a bronchus. Pus from the chest does not pass below the diaphragm into the abdomen. Inhaled vomit most commonly passes into the right lower lobe of the lungs.

A6.39
A. False
B. True
C. False
D. False
E. True

The Glasgow System classifies acute pancreatitis as severe if three of the following criteria are present:

- Age > 55 years
- White blood cell count > 15×10^9/l
- Blood glucose > 10 mmol/l
- Serum urea > 16 mmol/l
- Arterial oxygen saturation (PaO_2) < 60 mmol/l
- Serum calcium < 2.0 mmol/l
- Serum albumin < 32 g/l
- Lactate dehydrogenase > 600 u/l
- Aspartate aminotransferase or alanine aminotransferase > 100 IU/l

A6.40

A. True
B. True
C. True
D. True
E. False

Fatty liver is a recognised cause for right hypochondrial pain. Pancreatic pain is central and radiates to the back. In 10% of patients with peptic ulcer disease pain is referred to the right hypochondrium.

A6.41

A. True
B. True
C. True
D. True
E. True

All of these may be the cause of acute abdominal fluid collections. In cirrhosis there is often some added insult such as sepsis, alcoholic binges or development of hepatocellular carcinoma.

A6.42

A. True
B. False
C. True
D. True
E. True

Nitrates (and calcium antagonists) relax the oesophageal sphincter, aggravating reflux but sometimes helping oesophageal spasm or achalasia. Asacol releases mesalazine when pH rises in the distal ileum; this occurs too soon if gastric acid is suppressed. Domperidone (and metoclopramide) stimulate prolactin release and can result in mastalgia/galactorrhoea.

A6.43

A. True
B. True
C. True
D. False
E. False

A raised platelet count could be indicative of inflammatory bowel disease but also coeliac disease or blood loss. Hyposplenism is also associated with both coeliac disease and inflammatory bowel disease. Multiple stool cultures may fail to demonstrate giardiasis. Hypolactasia is a common secondary problem with coeliac disease.